FOUNDATION TO DENTAL CORE TRAINING

SECURING YOUR TOP TRAINING POST

Written with the UK's top 1% ranked Dental Core Trainees

DR KALPESH PRAJAPAT
DR DIMA MOBARAK

Printed in the United Kingdom. First Printing, 2018

Second Edition

ISBN: 978-17-95817-73-8

The information contained in this book reflects the views and opinions
of its individual contributors and authors, and is in no way intended to
be representative of COPDEND or associated official organisations.

While every effort has been made to ensure that this information is
reliable and accurate with respect to Dental Core Training recruitment,
it must be noted that this book is not an official document.

We would encourage all individuals wishing to partake in the Dental
Core Training recruitment process to seek official clarification and
advice from resources endorsed by COPDEND.

The sample scenarios and answers presented in this book are those
created by the contributors and authors, from their own anecdotal
clinical experiences, and are not designed to be rehearsed. Above all,
we would encourage all readers to use our guidelines to develop and
enhance their own approach to answering these questions.

We really hope this book adds value to your interview preparation by giving you first-hand insights of what to expect during the interview and a more in-depth understanding of what to expect from Dental Core Training.

All the best!

Table of Contents

Preface

Over the past few years, there has been increased interest in pursuing Dental Core Training.

For Dental Core Training 1 posts, this may be due to more young dentists wanting to develop further skills following Dental Foundation Training and possibly individuals not quite knowing what to do following their first year in practice. For those with existing Dental Core Trainee 1 or 2 posts, applying for an additional year of training may also be considered to help build experience in preparation for specialty training posts.

Dental Core Training recruitment, just like Foundation Training, is reliant upon the candidate ranking as highly as possible for them to be offered their desired training post. The process of recruitment becomes much more challenging during Dental Core Training owing to the limited number and variation of posts available.

This book is intended to be of interest to those considering applying for Dental Core Training 1, 2 and 3 posts, especially for those who may not know about the programme or the application process. By the end of this book, you should be more familiar with what DCT is, the benefits it will bring you, and how to go about securing a top rank in the challenging interview process.

Acknowledgements

We are extremely grateful to the Dental Core Trainees, specialist dentists and consultants who have contributed their anecdotal experience and knowledge towards making this resource more factual and valuable for our readers.

Special gratitude to our key contributors:

Dr. Vinay Chavda BSc (Hons), BDS (Hons), MJDF RCS (Eng), PGCert MedEd

Dr. Amit Dattani DMD, MFDS RCPS (Glasg)

Dr. Michael Santangeli BDS (Hons), BSc (Hons)

Dr. Natalie Bradley BDS, MFDS RCS (Edin)

Dr. Devan S Raindi BDS (Hons), MJDF RCS (Eng)

Dr. Satnam Singh Virdee BDS, MFDS RCS (Edin), PGCert DentEd

Dr. Rui Albuquerque DDS, MS, FHEA, PhD

Common Acronyms

Throughout Foundation Training you were likely to come across a plethora of acronyms relating to various dental terminology. Below is a list of common acronyms likely to be mentioned when discussing Dental Core Training.

ACS Advanced Card Systems

ADH Adult Dental Health

BDA British Dental Association

BSc Bachelor of Science

CBD Case Base Discussion

CDH Child Dental Health

COPDEND UK Committee of Postgraduate Deans and Directors

CPA Consumer Protection Act

CPD Continuing Professional Development

CQC Care Quality Commission

DCT Dental Core Training

DFT Dental Foundation Training

DMF Dental and Maxillofacial Radiology

DOP Direct Observation of Procedural Skills

EPR Electronic Patient Record

FD Foundation Dentist

GDC General Dental Council

GDP General Dental Practices

HEE Health Education England

HSCNI Health & Social Care Services in Northern Ireland

IOTN Index of Orthodontic Treatment Need

LEP local education provider

LETBs Local Education and Training Boards

LIMS Laboratory Information Management System

MDM Mobile Device Managers

MDT Multidisciplinary Team

MFDS Membership of the Faculty of Dental Surgery

MJDF Membership of the Joint Dental Faculties

Mini CEX Mini Clinical Evaluation Exercise

MSF NIMDTA Multisource Feedback Northern Ireland Medical and Dental Training Agency

NCAS National Clinical Assessment Service

NES NHS Education for Scotland

NICE National Institute for Health and Care Excellence

NPSA National Patient Safety Agency

OMFS Oral and Maxillofacial Surgery

PACS Picture Archiving and Communications System

PAR Peer Assessment Rating

PAT Peer Assessment Tool

PDP Personal Development Plan

PHE Public Health England

RCP Review of Competence Progression

SHO Senior House Officer

SIGN Scottish Intercollegiate Guidelines Network

SJT Situational Judgement Test

SLE Supervised Learning Event

SMART Specific, Measurable, Attainable, Relevant and Timely

TAB Team Assessment of Behaviours

TPD Training Programme Director

VT Dental Vocational Training

WBA Workplace Based Assessment

GDC Definitions of Dental Specialties

Many DCT posts will involve training within a specific dental specialty or even a rotation of two or more specialisms. The below list provides a brief description of each dental specialty in accordance with GDC definitions.

Special Care Dentistry: This is concerned with the improvement of the oral health of individuals and groups in society who have a physical, sensory, intellectual, mental, medical, emotional or social impairment or disability or, more often, a combination of these factors. It pertains to adolescents and adults.

Oral Surgery: This deals with the treatment and ongoing management of irregularities and pathologies of the jaw and mouth that require surgical intervention. This includes the specialty previously called Surgical Dentistry.

Orthodontics: This is the development, prevention, and correction of irregularities of the teeth, bite, and jaw.

Paediatric Dentistry: This is concerned with comprehensive therapeutic oral health care for children from birth through adolescence, including care for those who demonstrate intellectual, medical, physical, psychological and/or emotional problems.

Endodontics: This is concerned with the cause, diagnosis, prevention, and treatment of diseases and injuries of the tooth root, dental pulp, and surrounding tissue.

Periodontics: The diagnosis, treatment, and prevention of diseases and disorders (infections and inflammation) of the gums and other structures around the teeth.

Prosthodontics: The replacement of missing teeth and the associated soft and hard tissues by prostheses (crowns, bridges, dentures) which may be fixed or removable, or may be supported and retained by implants.

Restorative Dentistry: This deals with the restoration of diseased, injured, or abnormal teeth to normal function. This includes all aspects of Endodontics, Periodontics, and Prosthodontics.

Oral Medicine: Concerned with the oral health care of patients with chronic recurrent and medically related disorders of the mouth and with their diagnosis and non-surgical management.

Oral Microbiology: Diagnosis and assessment of facial infection – typically bacterial and fungal disease. This is a clinical specialty undertaken by laboratory-based personnel who provide reports and advice based on interpretation of microbiological samples.

Oral and Maxillofacial Pathology: Diagnosis and assessment made from tissue changes characteristic of disease of the oral cavity, jaws, and salivary glands. This is a clinical specialty undertaken within a laboratory environment.

Dental and Maxillofacial Radiology: Involves all aspects of medical imaging that provide information about anatomy, function, and diseased states of the teeth and jaws.

Oral and Maxillofacial Surgery: Involves the diagnosis and treatment of any disease affecting the mouth, jaws, face, and neck. This includes oral surgery (impacted teeth, dental cysts, dental implants, etc.), injuries to the face, salivary gland problems, cancers of the head and neck, facial deformity, oral medicine (ulcers, red/white patches, mouth cancer), facial pain and TMJ disorders.

Key Resources

Together with the team of contributors and authors, a list of key resources has been compiled to provide you with the essential reading material and guidance for preparation.

As always, preparation is vital, and a full understanding of the recruitment process is beneficial to put you ahead of the competition. Given you are reading this book, you are likely to be amongst the few who will have access to the insight from the past top-ranked DCT candidates.

Oriel http://www.oriel.nhs.uk

Oriel is the portal you will use for application for Dental Core Training posts and Specialist Training posts. Oriel is an online recruitment portal for postgraduate dental training posts.

Through Oriel you can register for training posts, browse and apply for post vacancies, book interviews, and manage posts and offers, and all communications will be received via Oriel's online messaging system.

COPDEND (Committee of Postgraduate Dental Deans and Directors) http://www.copdend.org/

COPDEND are responsible for the delivery of postgraduate education and training in primary and secondary care for the dental team. The committee includes all the postgraduate dental deans and directors in the UK. The recruitment, education, and development of Dental Core Training posts are also influenced by this committee.

Their website features official information required for DCT recruitment including post descriptions, DCT person specifications, and other essential information you must know.

COPDEND Silver Guide (published September 2018)

https://www.copdend.org/wp-content/uploads/2018/08/Dental-Silver-Guide-2018-Final-160818.pdf_

The COPDEND Silver Guide provides an essential overview of Dental Core Training in the UK. This document covers a range of information ranging from recruitment to the standards expected from the trainee. This comprehensive guidance is downloadable from the COPDEND website.

COPDEND Dental Gold Guide (Fourth Edition)

http://www.copdend.org//data/files/Dental Gold Guide/Dental Gold Guide June 2016 - updated FEB17.pdf

COPDEND have developed a comprehensive guide to postgraduate specialty training within the UK. The latest edition was completed June 2016 and can be downloaded from the above link.

DCT curriculum (Last updated 14/12/16)

http://www.copdend.org/data/files/Downloads/2016 12 14 UK DCT Curriculum - December 2016.pdf

The Dental Core Training curriculum has been developed by COPDEND to bring a structured framework to improve DCTs' educational outcomes. The curriculum aims to promote early postgraduate professional development through a competence framework which seeks to enhance the DCTs' skills, knowledge, and professional attributes to allow trainees to progress to various dental career aspirations.

Health Education England (HEE)

The aim of Health Education England (HEE) is to help improve patient care through the delivery of training and education to dentists throughout England. HEE work with local healthcare professionals such as doctors, dentists, and nurses and key stakeholders to improve outcomes and patient experience. The local deanery will support postgraduate education, workforce development, and the training of Dental Core Trainees.

Below is a list of the websites where more information can be found on each deanery:

- East Midlands https://www.eastmidlandsdeanery.nhs.uk/

  Areas included: Derbyshire, Leicestershire and Rutland, Lincolnshire, Northamptonshire, and Nottinghamshire

- East of England https://heeoe.hee.nhs.uk/dental_home
  Counties included: Essex, Bedfordshire, Hertfordshire, Cambridgeshire, Norfolk, and Suffolk

- Kent, Surrey, Sussex

  http://www.kssdeanery.ac.uk/dental

- North Central and London
  http://www.lpmde.ac.uk/training-programme/dental

- North East
  http://madeinheene.hee.nhs.uk/dental_training

- North West
  https://www.nwpgmd.nhs.uk/

- North West London
  http://www.lpmde.ac.uk/training-programme/dental

- London and South East
  http://www.lpmde.ac.uk/training-programme/dental

- South West
  http://www.dental.southwest.hee.nhs.uk/

  Areas included: Gloucestershire, Somerset, Devon, Cornwall, Wiltshire, and Dorset

- Thames Valley and Wessex
  http://www.oxforddeanery.nhs.uk/dental_school.aspx

  Areas include: Berkshire, Buckinghamshire and Milton Keynes, Oxfordshire, and Hampshire and the Isle of Wight

- Wessex operate through the Thames Valley and Wessex website above

- West Midlands
  https://www.westmidlandsdeanery.nhs.uk/Dentistry

- Yorkshire and Humber
  http://www.yorksandhumberdeanery.nhs.uk/dentistry/

NHS Education for Scotland (NES)

http://www.nes.scot.nhs.uk/education-and-training/by-discipline/dentistry.aspx

NES provides postgraduate education and training for dentists and other healthcare professionals. In Scotland NES functions as a special health board within NHS Scotland and is responsible for developing and delivering undergraduate, postgraduate, and continuing professional development and education within the regions of Edinburgh, Glasgow, Dundee, Aberdeen, and Inverness.

Dental Postgraduate Training and Education in Wales

https://dental.walesdeanery.org/homepage-dental

Funded through the Welsh government, the Wales deanery aims to improve the oral health of Wales through the provision of postgraduate education and training for Foundation Dentists (FD), Dental Core Trainees (DCT), Specialty Registrars (StR) and Dental Care Professionals (DCP).

Northern Ireland Medical and Dental Training Agency

http://www.nimdta.gov.uk/

NIMDTA supports and organises the training, recruitment, and continued professional development of healthcare professionals, including Dental Core Trainees. Their website also contains information about current DCT posts and locations.

Useful books

Medical Interviews (2nd Edition): A comprehensive guide to CT, ST & Registrar Interview Skills – Over 120 medical interview questions, techniques, and NHS topics explained

Author: Olivier Picard

This book was an overall essential read prior to the assessment centre. It provides factual and relevant questions with answers to typical medical/dental interview scenarios.

Oxford Assess and Progress: Situational Judgement Test

Author: David Metcalfe

This book is useful to practice SJTs under timed conditions and learn the techniques in which to save time and score highly. The book has medical SJTs, but the principles behind ranking the answers remain the same. The SJT assessment will involve scenarios based in hospital settings, including those where you act as an OMFS DCT, so it is essential to be familiar with the medical terminology.

On-call in Oral and Maxillofacial Surgery (2nd Edition)

Author: Karl F. B. Payne

An essential read for applicants who are not familiar with the management of maxillofacial scenarios. This is an easy-to-read, relevant book that will prepare applicants for the clinical scenario station.

Clinical Guidelines

Having a good basic understanding of the clinical guidelines will be useful for your role as a DCT. The clinical scenario and the clinical communication stations will require a basic knowledge of the guidelines in order to discuss and manage the cases presented. Not all of the guidelines below will be relevant during the assessment, but being aware that they exist is essential when you start DCT.

British Society of Periodontology (BSP)

- Basic Periodontal Exam (BPE) 2016

- Referral policy and parameters of care 2011

- Guidelines for periodontal screening and management of children and adolescents under 18 years of age. Guidelines produced in conjunction with the British Society of Periodontology and British Society of Paediatric Dentistry 2012

- The Good Practitioner's Guide to Periodontology 2016 (3rd edition)

British Endodontic Society (BES)

- European Society of Endodontology position statement: The use of CBCT in endodontics

- Quality guidelines for endodontic treatment: consensus report of the European Society of Endodontology

British Society for the Study of Prosthetics in Dentistry (BSSPD)

- Guides to Standards in Prosthetic Dentistry – Complete and Partial Dentures

- Guidelines on Standards for the Treatment of Patients using Endosseous Implants

- Prosthetic Dentistry Glossary (Revision 1995)

British Society for Restorative Dentistry (BSRD)

- Crown, bridge and implant guidelines

British Society for Oral Medicine

- Common Oral Medicine patient information leaflets will be useful to read to understand how to communicate common oral medicine conditions in lay terms to patients.

British Society for Disability and Oral Health

- Multi-disciplinary Guidelines for the Oral Management of Patients following Oncology Treatment updated 2012

- Clinical Guidelines & Integrated Care Pathways for the Oral Health Care of People with Learning Disabilities updated 2012

- Guidelines for the Delivery of a Domiciliary Oral Health-care Service revised 2009

- The Provision of Oral Care under General Anaesthesia in Special Care Dentistry – A Professional Consensus Statement, 2009

- Principles on Intervention for People Unable to Comply with Routine Dental Care

- Guidelines for Oral Health Care for Long-stay Patients and Residents

- Guidelines for the Development of Local Standards of Oral Health Care for Dependent, Dysphagic, Critically and Terminally Ill Patients

- Oral Health Care for People with Mental Health Problems

- Guidelines for Oral Health Care for People with a Physical Disability

British Society of Paediatric Dentistry (BSPD)

- Guidelines for Periodontal Screening and Management of Children and Adolescents (2012)

- Management and Root Canal Treatment of Non-Vital Immature Permanent Incisor Teeth (2010)

- Non-Pharmacological Behaviour Management (Revised 2011)

- Treatment of Avulsed Permanent Incisor Teeth in Children (Peter Day. Revised 2012)

- Guidelines for the Management of Children Referred for Dental Extraction under General Anaesthesia (August 2011)

National Institute for Health and Care Excellence (NICE)

- Prophylaxis against infective endocarditis: Antimicrobial prophylaxis against infective endocarditis in adults and children undergoing interventional procedures

- Dental checks: intervals between oral health reviews

- Guidance on the Extraction of Wisdom Teeth

- Service guidance on improving outcomes in head and neck cancers

- Suspected cancer: recognition and referral

Faculty of General Dental Practitioners (FGDP)

- Selection Criteria for Dental Radiography

- Dementia-Friendly Dentistry

- Clinical Examination and Record-Keeping

- Antimicrobial Prescribing for GDPs

Scottish Dental Clinical Effectiveness Programme (SDCEP)

- Oral Health Management of Patients at Risk of Medication-related Osteonecrosis of the Jaw – updated March 2017

- Conscious sedation in dentistry – updated June 2012

- Decontamination into practice – updated Oct 2014

- Prevention and Management of Dental Caries in Children – April 2010

- Drug prescribing for dentistry – updated Jan 2016

- Emergency Dental Care – updated Nov 2013

- Management of dental patients taking anticoagulants or antiplatelet drugs – Aug 2015

- Management of Acute Dental Problems – March 2013

- Oral Health Assessment and Review – March 2011

- Oral health management of patients prescribed bisphosphonates – April 2011

- Prevention and treatment of periodontal disease in primary care – June 2014

International Association of Dental Trauma (IADT)

- Dental trauma guidelines (revised 2012)

Royal College of Surgeons England (RCS)

- Management of Unerupted Maxillary Incisors (2016)

- Management of the Palatally Ectopic Maxillary Canine (2016)

- Guideline for the Extraction of First Permanent Molars in Children (2014)

- Temporomandibular Disorders (TMDs): an update and management guidance for primary care from the UK Specialist Interest Group in Orofacial Pain and TMDs (USOT) (2013)

- Diagnosis, Prevention, and Management of Dental Erosion (2013)

- The Oral Management of Oncology Patients Requiring Radiotherapy, Chemotherapy and/or Bone Marrow Transplantation (2012)

- Guidelines for Selecting Appropriate Patients to Receive Treatment with Dental Implants: Priorities for the NHS (2012)

- Guidelines for Surgical Endodontics 2012

- Clinical Guidelines and Integrated Care Pathways for the Oral Health Care of People with Learning Disabilities 2012

- Pulp Therapy for Primary Molars (2006)

- Extraction of Primary Teeth – Balance And Compensation (2006)

- The Management of Patients with Third Molar Teeth (2006 but under review)

- Managing Anxious Children: the Use of Conscious Sedation in Paediatric Dentistry (2002)

- Restorative Dentistry: Index of Treatment Need – Complexity Assessment (2001)

- Management of Pericoronitis (reviewed 2004)

- Management and Prevention of Dry Socket (reviewed 2004)

- Management of Unilateral Fractures of the Condyle (reviewed 2000)

Scottish Intercollegiate Guidelines Network (SIGN)

- Diagnosis and management of head and neck cancer – SIGN 90

- Management of Unerupted and Impacted Third Molar Teeth – SIGN 43

- Dental interventions to prevent caries in children – SIGN 138

- Prevention and management of dental decay in the pre-school child

- Preventing Dental Caries in Children at High Caries Risk

NHS Health Protection Agency

- Guidance on the Safe Use of Dental Cone Beam Computed Tomography (CBCT)

European Commission

- Guidelines on CBCT for Dental and Maxillofacial Radiology

Legislation

- GDC Standards for the Dental Team 2013

- Principles of Ethical Advertising 2012

- Medicines and Healthcare Product Regulatory 2014

- Access to Health Records Act 1990

- Care Quality Commission (Registration) Regulations 2009

- Health and Social Care Act 2008 (Regulated Activities) Regulations 2014

- Bolam Test and Montgomery Law

- Mental Capacity Act 2005

- Data Protection Act 1998

- Family Law Reform Act 1969

- Age of Legal Capacity (Scotland) Act 1991

- Gillick/Fraser competency

- Children Act 1989

- Consumer Protection Act 1998

- Dentist Act 1984

Pay Circulars (Medical & Dental)
http://www.nhsemployer.org

For more information regarding DCT salary, you should refer to the Pay Circulars (Medical & Dental) published by NHS employers. DCTs who have on-call commitments and those based in the London deaneries will get additional salary weighting.

Dates for 2019 applications

Table 1 describes the key dates you should pencil into your diary. These dates are available on the COPDEND website and apply to DCT 1, 2 and 3 posts.

Table 1. Key Dates for 2019 DCT 1,2 & 3 Applications

Key milestones	Explanation	Dates for 2019
DCT advert appears	The DCT job advert appears on Oriel website (but the application cannot be submitted). A good time to read the DCT National Person Specification 2019.	15/1/19
Application opens	The DCT application opens; you can begin to fill out the generic application form to be considered for longlisting.	22/1/19
Advert and application close	You must submit your completed application by this date otherwise you will NOT be eligible for a DCT post for 2019.	12/2/19
SJT invites sent out (6pm GMT)	The date you will be sent an invitation to book an SJT time slot for the date you will sit the SJT.	11/3/19
SJT assessment window	The SJT examination will be conducted on one of these days within the range, based on your preference.	20/3/19– 27/3/19
Selection centre invite sent (6pm GMT)	The date you will be sent an invitation to book your selection centre interview, which will be the date you attend for assessment.	2/4/19
Selection centre booking deadline (6pm GMT)	This is the deadline for booking your selection centre. All places are first come first served, so book early!	5/4/19
Selection centre assessment window	The national assessments will be conducted throughout these dates. Therefore, the time you attend for assessment will be on one of these dates.	29/4/19– 3/5/19
First offers released	The first day that job offers for DCT posts will be announced.	20/5/19

Key milestones	Explanation	Dates for 2019
Holding deadline	This is the date by which all held offers must have a decision made (accept or reject).	13/6/19
Upgrading deadline	The date up to which a higher preferenced post may be offered to you (if you have opted into upgrades on Oriel after receiving an offer which is not your first choice).	20/6/19
Final iteration of offers	This is the date that all final offers will be made. No further offers will be made after this date.	21/6/19
Paperwork deadline	This is the date that your paperwork must be submitted for completion of employment checks.	28/6/19

Changes from 2018 applications

Below are some of the critical changes to Dental Core Training applications since the 2018 recruitment process. This section will be useful for those who applied for 2018 posts and are considering re-applying, and for those considering DCT 2 and 3 posts.

1) Since the 2017 recruitment round, the SJT (Situational Judgement Test) now falls on a separate date to the station assessments.

    The dates for which you may select your SJT assessment in 2019 are: Wednesday 20th March – Wednesday 27th March 2019. The SJT is now conducted as a computer-based assessment, at a Pearson VUE test centre. Previously this was sat following the station assessments at the selection centre, on the same day.

    For the SJT assessment, you will be required to book this when invites are sent out. For 2019 these invites will be sent on Monday 11th March 2019 at 6pm.

    Importantly, this differs from the 2018 round, where the invite was not sent at a specific time. It is worth mentioning that the SJT locations (Pearson VUE test centres) do get booked on a first-come, first-served basis. As such, it is crucial to act promptly in order to secure your SJT centre of choice.

A tutorial of how to use this computer-based system can be found online at http://www.pearsonvue.com/athena/.

2) For DCT 2 and 3 applicants, the portfolio station was previously a station where your portfolio would be assessed, without you being present. (Your portfolio would be taken from you at the registration stage, at the start of the assessment day, and handed to independent assessors for review, then returned to you after you had completed all the stations).

Assessment of your portfolio would often involve two independent assessors scoring your portfolio against a pre-defined score sheet, taking into consideration your own 'self-assessment score' – this being your self-critical score of your individual portfolio. Full details on creating the portfolio, including a step-by-step guide to producing this, will be discussed in Chapter 4.

For 2019, the portfolio station (for DCT 2 and 3 applicants) will now involve the applicant discussing and answering questions about their portfolio in front of this panel of assessors. This, therefore, will be treated as an additional station. This will provide opportunities for the applicant to elaborate on key aspects of their portfolio. For full details on this change please see the COPDEND website. http://www.copdend.org/

Chapter 1

DCT: Why, What, Where and When?

So what is DCT?

Dental Core Training (DCT) is a training pathway for postgraduate dentists. DCT has been renamed over the last five years from Senior House Office (SHO) to Dental Foundation Year 2 (DFT 2) to Career Development Posts (CDP) to now DCT.

DCT is a structured pathway and typically occurs following Foundation Training. For some, this is the stepping-stone to specialty training (StR). For others, it may be an additional period of training to enhance or learn valuable practical competencies for exit into primary dental care (General Dental Service, Community Dental Services or Public Dental Services) or secondary care posts such as Specialty Dentist roles. The purpose of DCT is to enable recent dental graduates an opportunity to gain additional skills and competencies in particular dental specialisms.

DCT is a not a mandatory requirement for Foundation Dentists, but provides various benefits, which are discussed below. DCT 1 posts are held for 12 months, and the training ranges from 1 to 3 years, meaning there is no Dental Core Training post beyond DCT 3.

Following appointment to each 12-month post, a trainee must re-apply to be considered for a subsequent year of training. So, following DCT 1, trainees must go through national recruitment again to apply for DCT 2 posts.

DCT is a salaried training post, and there are limited numbers of intake per year. The cost of training is partly paid by Health Education England and partly by the employing NHS trust. Therefore, entry to DCT is highly competitive.

The DCT programme has a formal curriculum, and DCTs are expected to achieve mandatory outcomes. There are a variety of DCT training posts, with some roles having only one or two spaces. Each post will focus on training through the workplace, and therefore, trainees provide service within primary or secondary care during their post.

DCT year 1 (which usually follows Dental Foundation Training (DFT)) will focus on generic outcomes, rather than concentrating on specific 'procedure'-based outcomes; it is aimed at improving general skills to a competent level. DCT years 2 and 3 (which follow DCT year 1 or 2 respectively) will focus on further development of these generic skills. DCT 2 and 3s will develop additional competencies beyond the level of a general practitioner, with DCT 2s gaining experience of specialist skills and DCT 3s enhancing specialist skills. Development of these skills and experience may better prepare trainees for entry into specialist training pathways. For the full list of outcomes you can expect following DCT training, please refer to the COPDEND DCT curriculum (see Key Resources).

Each DCT will be assigned an educational supervisor, and trainees will agree on a personal development plan (PDP) with their educational supervisor at the beginning of a training period, the aim of which is to stimulate self-directed learning.

Like DFT, the DCT will use an online portfolio to collate evidence of training and supervised learning events including direct observation of procedure skills, case-based discussion, developing the clinical tutor, mini clinical evaluation exercises (mini-CEX) and reflections. It is estimated that two supervised learning events (as mentioned above) should be undertaken per month. Trainees are able to set personal targets and evidence their progression through these events and ultimately improve clinical development to the level of an advanced practitioner.

At the end of each training period, the trainee's progress is reviewed through a formal review of clinical progression, and a certificate of achievement is awarded.

What happens after DCT 3?

The DCT programme is for a maximum of three years only. Beyond Dental Core Training Year 3, trainees may develop additional skills or experience through specialty training (StR) or service posts, e.g. Trust Specialty Dentist/Staff Grade. Alternatively, a DCT may decide to pursue general practice with an additional interest in their particular field of training.

Following any level of exit from DCT, trainees are likely to have additional competencies developed beyond those in DFT and have many career options available (Figure 2 in Chapter 5).

Why do it?

The DCT programme has a number of benefits following foundation training, including clarification of dental career plans and enhancement of core skills.

Enabling this is the DCT curriculum, which provides a structured framework so that trainees may pursue early career progression. This also guides trainees to acquire enhanced skill sets and evidence outcomes through the e-portfolio.

Benefits:

- Exposure to a variety of clinical environments provides beneficial clinical and educational experience for those early on in their dental career
- Experience within different dental settings and working with various clinicians allows better understanding and clarity over which career pathway to take
- Compared to DFT, DCTs have the opportunity to work in a varied environment, with different patient types, and undertake a variety of treatments
- DCTs work with the support of senior clinicians, where they have access to assistance and supervision
- DCTs are able to learn through experience and treatment of NHS patients within a safe environment
- DCTs can practise with sufficient feedback and supervision to allow development of existing skills, subsequently leading to the acquisition of additional skill sets
- DCTs can learn from colleagues who have varying levels of experience and backgrounds in different settings
- DCTs can learn to manage patients in secondary care who have been referred from practitioners in primary dental care
- DCTs have the opportunity to understand, manage, and treat complex dental conditions
- DCTs get to manage and treat patients with complex medical conditions, including complex mental health/psychiatric conditions, and those with both complex medical and dental conditions
- DCTs gain experience of working within a multidisciplinary team
- DCTs can undertake activities which may impact on the operation of a service, including clinical and organisational governance such as service evaluation, clinical audit or research
- DCTs have the opportunity to discuss cases and work alongside consultants and academic specialists

- DCTs can be part of projects and activities that are supported by large organisations, such as teaching hospital study groups, lectures or tutorials
- DCTs can get involved in teaching undergraduates
- As a DCT, you will be surrounded by like-minded individuals and colleagues who are likely to have pursued a pathway you may wish to take
- DCTs have the opportunity to showcase skills they have developed, at presentation days and national conferences, and gain awards for recognition
- DCTs can learn many new clinical skills
- After completing DCT, you will have an evidenced portfolio of skills and outcomes you have achieved to demonstrate to future employers
- DCTs can develop enhanced skills to open different career pathway options

Drawbacks

- There is a competitive application process
- You may not achieve the desired post you want
- Posts may have on-call requirements (but OMFS posts are higher paid due to this)
- Posts may include elements of specialisms that you have no interest in
- You are required to maintain an updated e-portfolio of learning events
- There are elements of administrative tasks such as dictating letters and writing reports
- Some posts only have a short rotation within a given specialty, e.g. general duties posts or posts which switch after 6 months
- Compared to associate dentists with a similar level of experience, DCTs may work more hours but be remunerated at a lower rate.

What does the job involve?

Types of posts

Most DCT posts across the UK are in Oral and Maxillofacial Surgery (OMFS) Units in District General Hospitals and University Teaching Hospitals. A smaller number of positions are available within Dental Teaching Hospitals, with the remainder in the salaried/public dental service and General Dental Practices (GDP) with specialist input.

Currently, the majority of dentistry is carried out in primary care dental practices on the high street, in community dental services, or in specialist clinics under GDS (General Dental Services) or PDS (Personal Dental Service) contracts.

However, the majority of specialist dental services are provided via acute hospitals, NHS trusts, District General Hospitals, and University Teaching Hospitals, and it is here that DCTs will be based to ensure service delivery and learn through practice.

Generic job description and duties of posts

(Please note that all posts differ; therefore, you should refer to the COPDEND website for accurate job descriptions.)

Oral and maxillofacial surgery

The OMFS DCT will gain experience in the management of oral and maxillofacial diseases and conditions including facial deformities, salivary gland surgery, trauma, dental infections, oral medicine and TMJPDS. There will be opportunities to acquire and develop skills and improve current oral surgery experience through supervised MOS.

DCTs will gain experience through observation and assistance during head and neck oncology cases, orthognathic treatments and trauma cases. Also, OMFS DCTs will attend new outpatient clinics and gain knowledge in treatment planning and diagnosis. Consultant-led outpatient clinics deal with managing oral surgery, and maxillofacial and oral medicine-related referrals.

Typical staff amongst the OMFS team include:

Consultant Oral and Maxillofacial Surgeons, Consultant Orthodontists, Consultant Restorative Dental Surgeon, Staff Grade Doctors and Specialist Registrars.

Community dentistry

Some posts may involve a rotation within Community Dental Services. This involves working within the various aspects of the community service, complex special care, paediatrics, and working with hard-to-reach patients, as well as urgent care and drop-in services. It may also involve working in different clinics, domiciliary care, and possibly working on the mobile unit and GA within theatre. The post offers a wide range of experiences treating patients who are vulnerable and require extra support to enable dental care to be carried out.

Restorative dentistry

DCTs in restorative dentistry may attend consultant-led new patient clinics and multidisciplinary clinics. DCTs are likely to undertake a wide range of restorative treatments including periodontal treatment, endodontics, fixed and removable prosthodontics, conservative dentistry, and prevention.

DCTs may undertake treatment clinics in Special Care and emergency dental services.

Oral surgery

In oral surgery, DCTs are likely to experience the full scope and range of outpatient oral surgery, with supervision according to their individual needs. They may also participate in treatment under LA and IV sedation in the Oral Surgery department and may also manage patients in the primary care/emergency department.

DCT may also assist with the outpatient consultant clinics, MDT clinics, and consultant treatment sessions.

Paediatric dentistry

In paediatric dentistry, DCTs may attend consultant-led new patient clinics and MDT clinics. DCTs are likely to undertake a wide range of treatments for children and are likely to experience the management of complex medical histories and behaviour management in children, including inhalation sedation.

Orthodontics

In orthodontics, DCTs are likely to attend consultant-led new patient clinics and MDT clinics. DCTs may be involved in the assessment of new orthodontic patients and present findings to the consultant to help with developing treatment plans. DCT may be involved in undertaking treatment such as bonding brackets or changing wires in consultant-led treatment sessions. It is worth noting that this specialty is usually experienced as a mixed post rather than an entire 12-month period in orthodontics.

General duties posts

General duties posts tend to encompass a number of specialities whereby the DCT will rotate amongst the different specialisms throughout their 12-month training post. An example of a DCT 1 general duties rota could include: acute dental clinic, oral surgery with intravenous sedation or local anaesthesia, periodontal treatments, restorative treatments, oral medicine, and paediatric clinics. The exact job descriptions between trusts and hospitals will vary, so it is important to read the job description carefully on COPDEND.

Mixed posts, e.g. restorative/oral surgery or paediatrics/OMFS

Certain DCT posts will have an element of more than one specialty but differ from general duties in that the DCT will likely be limited to two specialties. These positions may occur over a 6-month rotation period, where the DCT will spend 6 months in one specialty and then rotate to their other specialty, or occur as a mixture of experience in their chosen specialities over the entire 12-month training period.

Where can I work?

There are a number of UK dental hospitals that currently provide teaching to undergraduates and postgraduates. DCT posts are available in dental hospitals, University Teaching Hospitals (UTH) and District General Hospitals (DGH). The typical job description will vary with trust, unit, and post; however, each facility will provide a range of services including:

1) Consultant advice, treatment planning, and treatment of patients referred by General Dental Practitioners and General Medical Practitioners

2) General dental treatments of patients for postgraduate/ undergraduate teaching purposes

3) Emergency dental care for acute trauma, pain, or dental disease

4) Treatment of outpatients or inpatients (DGH/UTH) where medical health conditions make it appropriate for their treatment to be conducted within the hospital

5) Dental treatments of short-stay patients or long-stay hospitals in patients (DGH/UTH)

These treatments include oral and maxillofacial surgery, oral surgery, orthodontics, paediatrics, and restorative dentistry.

A full list of post descriptions for DCT 1,2 and 3 posts, including their location, for 2019 will be available on the COPDEND website.

The British Association of Oral and Maxillofacial Surgeons (BAOMS) and the Committee of Postgraduate Dental Deans and Directors (COPDEND) have compiled a document that outlines guidelines for training of Dental Core Trainees (DCT) in OMFS Units: http://www.nes.scot.nhs.uk/media/4013444/DCTs in Hospitals.pdf

Amongst the posts that are available, it is worth researching the local deanery, possibly speaking to existing DCTs in that region, and looking carefully at the post description, noting the experiences you will gain and the hours of work.

Chapter 2

The Assessment Process

Eligibility

You must first study the DCT Person Specification Criteria which is available on the COPDEND website. This outlines exactly the requirements for DCT 1, 2 and 3 posts.

http://www.copdend.org/content.aspx?Group=foundation&Page=dct%202017%20recruitment

Each application will first be assessed via a national, systematic process, and those applicants who meet the criteria (outlined in the Person Specification) will be longlisted. Longlisting assures those applicants who fit the criteria a guaranteed interview slot at a selection centre.

TIP: You are advised that once selection centre preferencing is open, slots for interview bookings are taken on a first-come, first-served basis. So although you are guaranteed an interview slot, this may not be at your local selection centre, and you may need to travel further to an interview centre with an available interview slot.

Fret not, as selection is via national recruitment where all centres are standardised. It is worth noting, however, that dates differ between centres. Please see the COPDEND website for details on dates for each selection centre.

If you have any questions related to your eligibility, you should contact the applicant support service run by Dental Core Training National Office (DCTNO).

Dates for 2019

As Oriel will not consider any applications made beyond the deadline, it is strongly advised that all prospective DCTs familiarise themselves with the application process and be conscious of the dates. Table 1 (see Key Resources) shows the key dates for DCT in 2019.

The application process

All DCT posts are obtained via national recruitment, which has previously been coordinated by Health Education England's West Midlands Office. This process begins by completing an online application form via Oriel. Oriel has an applicant's user guide that provides help with the technical aspects of the online process; this can be found at https://www.oriel.nhs.uk/Web/ResourceBank/Edit/MQ==.

You will be required to complete a single online application form to apply for available posts within the 13 HEE (Health Education England) local offices, NES (NHS Education for Scotland), NIMDTA (Northern Ireland Dental and Training Agency) and the Wales deanery.

The application form has a similar layout to the DFT application form on Oriel, with generic questions and other dentistry-related questions such as qualifications, previous employment, and character references. It is essential you complete this accurately as changes may not be made after submission.

Following Oriel receiving your application, a systematic, standardised approach of longlisting will be completed, and all eligible applicants will be invited to book a place at a selection centre at a preferred location.

For the 2019 recruitment process, you will need to initially choose a centre for your SJT assessment and then subsequently another location for the selection centre in order to be appointed to a DCT programme. You must complete the SJT before progressing to the selection centre assessments.

How am I assessed?

Selection for DCT posts is based on national recruitment, similar to the recruitment for DFT posts. Selection is competitive, with entry criteria and assessment based on the DCT person specification.

In 2017, nearly 1 in 2 applicants were rejected due to high competition for DCT 1 posts.

Official 2017 statistics (Table 2) show that there were almost double the number of applicants to DCT 1 posts last year. In 2018, there were approximately 700 DCT posts (this included DCT 1, 2, and 3 posts).

Table 2. Official 2017 DCT statistics

Post	Applicants	Posts available	Reject rate (%)
DCT 1	663	384	42.1
DCT 2	375	223	40.5
DCT 3	159	57	64.2

Once you have completed the SJT and accepted your invitation to attend a selection centre, a structured assessment is conducted.

The format of the assessment consists of three stations for DCT 1 posts and an additional station for DCT 2 and 3 posts:

1) Clinical scenario

2) Clinical governance and risk management

3) Communication skills (with simulated patient who is an actor)

4) Portfolio assessment (DCT 2 and 3 posts)

Each element of the DCT assessment will allow you to demonstrate your compatibility and commitment to the DCT programme. In particular, assessors will be scoring you based on the 2019 DCT 1, 2 and 3 person specifications, depending whether you are applying for a DCT 1, 2 or 3 position. Specific criteria that cannot be demonstrated at the selection centre will be assessed using your references or your application form submitted through Oriel.

During the assessment, there will be four overarching criteria that will be evaluated by assessors:

1) Clinical skills – clinical knowledge & expertise

2) Personal skills

3) Probity – professional integrity

4) Commitment to learning and personal development

These categories can be further divided into essential or desirable criteria. Individuals who can demonstrate desirable characteristics stand a higher chance of achieving a better ranking than those without.

Essential criteria for Dental Core Training posts (adapted from the DCT National Person Specification)

Clinical skills – clinical knowledge & expertise

Capacity to apply sound clinical knowledge and awareness to full investigation of problems.

Assessors will want you to demonstrate a pragmatic approach to solving clinical problems with justification and reasoning. A good underlying knowledge of the clinical dilemma is required to manage a clinical scenario appropriately.

It is imperative to know that patient safety is paramount during DCT, so you should answer a question as a DCT 1, 2 or 3 depending on which post you are applying for. Knowing your own clinical capability and when to ask for help is crucial.

You will be able to demonstrate your understanding of clinical knowledge during the clinical scenario and clinical communication stations (described below).

Ability to conduct operating procedures

Assessors are likely to base this upon satisfactory completion of Foundation Training and your references. It is important to note that the assessors may access your DFT portfolio to view clinical data from Foundation Training.

Experience of clinical governance including clinical audit or significant event analysis

Clinical governance and risk management are elements of dentistry that aim to improve patient safety, clinical efficiency, and overall quality of patient care.

It is essential that you have had prior experience of clinical audit and significant event analysis and are able to discuss your own personal experience of undertaking such activities. You are likely to be assessed on these topics via the application form and during the clinical governance station.

Understanding of the principles and relevance of clinical research

An understanding of evidenced-based dentistry and clinical research is essential for prospective DCTs. Although you are not expected to have undertaken research, showing enthusiasm and a commitment to be involved in research is a desirable characteristic. This will be assessed on the application form and during the clinical governance station.

Personal skills

Evidence of personal skills will be assessed through the evidence on your application form, through your character references and based on your performance at the selection centre.

Characteristics of personal skills that are essential for the DCT applicant include:

Communication skills

You are expected to be an effective communicator with proficient oral and written English skills. The ability to be versatile and adaptable depending on the clinical situation is also essential.

Body language and tone of voice play a huge role in communication. You should aim to adapt your style of communication for the scenario, where you may have to show empathy and compassion.

Conceptual thinking and problem solving

You should show creativity and pragmatic thinking to resolve situations practically and with the patient's best interest in mind.

For the communication station, your aim is to make sure you solve the patients' concerns and ensure that they are listened to. It is important to have a logical and stepwise approach to managing challenging situations; often using the acronym SPIES can be helpful.

Seek further information about the clinical dilemma or scenario, put *patient* interest first by being proactive and considering patient safety, quality of care, and clinical efficiency. Aim to use your *initiative* to help manage the situation by delegating tasks or stepping in to help; following managing the initial clinical situation, aim to *escalate* the issue appropriately to a senior colleague, such as Clinical/Educational Supervisor, Duty Officer, Consultant, Clinical Lead, or Clinical Director. *Escalating* the issue aims to bring attention to others and so everyone can learn from the event. *Support* patients, colleagues, and staff to promote an 'everyone counts' attitude by providing help to prevent similar issues reoccurring; this should aim to be done confidentially and respectfully to those involved.

Empathy and sensitivity

You must be able to demonstrate a patient-centred approach and work respectfully with others.

Working within healthcare is one of the most sensitive and personal aspects of anyone's life; therefore, you must reflect this in your behaviour and communication with the patient.

Teamwork and leadership

You must show evidence of leadership and the ability to work with others within a team environment.

Teamwork encompasses the ability to work with others towards a common goal whilst also being able to act independently without continual assistance.

Demonstrating previous experience of this such as committee roles, projects you have been involved in, and contributions to team meetings would be well regarded. Also, to demonstrate leadership, it is important you share when you have identified a problem and implemented a change through working with people and evidencing this with real results. This could be an audit idea that came from a problem you observed or an issue you highlighted at a meeting and subsequently helped to fix.

Organisation and planning

You must demonstrate effective planning and organisational skills to meet deadlines and complete tasks.

Examples of organisational skills will often overlap with those of being a good team player and leader, and being professional. It is essential to be able to demonstrate these skills through activities you have undertaken during undergraduate or during postgraduate training. For example, in order to be more prepared for your day, you may attend clinics 15 minutes early to read through your schedule and make a list of equipment so your nurse can set this up prior to the patient arriving.

Coping with pressure

You must demonstrate the ability to cope in stressful situations and be capable of knowing when to seek advice to prevent putting patients at risk of harm. In the assessments, you may be asked about something you may not have seen or done before such as a maxillofacial scenario. It is important to be versatile and apply the same principles to each situation; when unsure, you should always suggest that you could always approach a senior colleague to reassure the examiner or patient that you are doing everything you can to help.

Values

You will be expected to demonstrate the NHS core values: Everyone counts, improving lives, commitment to quality of care, respect and dignity, working together for patients, and compassion.

Values will be evident in your behaviour, language, and communication. It is important you always remain professional despite facing a difficult patient or stern examiners. In order to display core values, remember to show respect for the entire team, consider the quality of patient care, and act safely.

Probity – professional integrity

The General Medical Council defines probity as being honest, trustworthy, and acting with integrity.

As a prospective DCT, you must demonstrate these characteristics throughout the assessment. In particular, the assessors will look to see if you show a professional attitude and respect for all, take responsibility for your actions, and show accountability.

It is therefore essential that you treat the assessment process as a formal matter, ensuring you are smartly dressed, timely, and courteous.

Commitment to learning and personal development

As mentioned earlier, DCT has many benefits and provides various career options. It is essential for you to be able to demonstrate an understanding of the prospective training post, its benefits, and how it will add value to your current skill set. In addition, you must show a desire to learn and develop skills and knowledge. This may be evidenced by a solid understanding of the DCT structure and the positive effect this will have on your career pathway. Furthermore, if you can show evidence of teaching, publication, presentation, awards, and desire for a postgraduate qualification, this will be positively favoured, as these are desirable characteristics for DCT applicants.

The selection centre

At the selection centre, you will have several opportunities to demonstrate how you fit the criteria outlined within the DCT National Person Specification.

The assessments include a series of question and role-play stations that are undertaken by trained dental professionals and actors.

These stations are akin to OSCEs and are conducted in formal timed conditions. Prior to the stations, on the day, you will be given a short overview and description of what to expect and how the stations are conducted, such as when to enter the rooms, and how the process will be performed. For those who attended UK Dental Foundation Training interviews, this will be a very similar process.

For the DCT 1 assessments, there will be three stations:

1) Clinical scenario

2) Clinical governance and risk management

3) Communication skills (with simulated patient who is an actor)

4) DCT 2 and 3 applicants will have an additional portfolio station (more details on the dental portfolio can be found on the COPDEND website and Chapter 4)

In order to best prepare yourself for these scenarios, we have collated realistic questions and formulated model answers with the aid of past top-ranking Dental Core Trainees and current Specialty Registrars.

1 The clinical scenario

What is this?

This station will involve a scenario that poses an issue which could be related to a mixture of both medical/dental related situations and clinical governance:

• Medically compromised patient

• Dental trauma: dentoalveolar/paediatrics

• Maxillofacial trauma: fractured zygoma/mandible

• Safeguarding

• Professionalism

• Raising concerns: hospital hierarchy

- Spreading infection and sepsis

- ABCDE and emergencies

- Working as a team: Liaising with other specialties

- Consent and capacity

What is expected of you?

You will come across clinical scenarios that you may not be familiar with, such as maxillofacial based scenarios. Do not change your approach! The examiners are looking for:

- A clear and structured approach

- Ability to identify key issues

- Ability to prioritise clinical needs (ABCDE approach)

- Awareness of your limitations

- Coping under pressure

You will be expected to:

- Take a clear and detailed history of the patient

- Systematically assess the patient

- Arrange appropriate investigations (blood tests, imaging, biopsy)

- Involve opinion from a senior colleague

- Construct a short-term management plan

- Be able to give an idea of a long-term plan

- Ensure all GDC principles are addressed

Despite only being dentally qualified and having had little experience in a hospital, you will still be expected to answer OMFS scenarios. The examiners are looking to see that you can apply principles you have learnt at undergraduate level, and that you have the initiative to answer these scenarios and practice safely within your competence.

How long do I get?

In previous years, 3 minutes has been given beforehand to read the scenario (which will usually be face down under the chair outside of the room). You are not allowed to write notes, but should read the brief clearly and understand what questions you should answer; usually, there are 3 to 4 questions. Following this, you will be asked to enter the room, where you will begin by speaking to the panel of assessors.

In previous years, this station has been 10 minutes, where the assessors usually begin by asking questions from a predetermined list. These questions are related to the scenario and often lead on in a logical sequence. A buzzer may be heard 1 minute prior to the end of the station.

Who will examine you?

You will typically have two examiners, who may be:

- Maxillofacial consultants

- Clinicians and consultants from a dental hospital

They may also be current educational supervisors in a secondary care setting, current postgraduate deans, and other members of the deanery.

COPDEND will provide assessors with a fixed mark scheme that will be given to all assessors throughout the UK. Therefore, it is likely that the assessors will be looking down at this during your assessment, so don't let this put you off.

Example of the DCT clinical scenario

You have 3 minutes to read this scenario.

You are a DCT working in a busy OMFS unit. It is 2am, and a 40-year-old male patient has presented with an injury to his face. He has significant periorbital swelling and bruising to the left side of his face localised to around his left eye. The patient attended alone and is English speaking but is worried about the swelling and pain. You are one of the first clinicians to see this patient.

Questions asked by assessors:

What would your initial assessment entail?

Confirm name and DOB. ABCDE approach to the patient. After having systematically covered an ABCDE assessment then assess injuries in detail. Life, limb, or sight injuries should be prioritised.

Note:

- D – 'Disability' may come in the form of alcohol intoxication; however, it is essential to rule out any cognitive disability as a result of head injury.

- Injuries involving the orbit must be carefully assessed for visual acuity/impairment. Never miss a retrobulbar haemorrhage!

History taking:

CO – Pain? Swelling? Funny bite? Numbness? Broken teeth? Facial weakness?

HPC

- Description of trauma and force of injury: Interpersonal violence? Foreign object (knuckle duster, tetanus risk)? Road traffic accident (wearing seatbelt, car vs. pedestrian)? Sporting injury?

- Any other injuries? Any signs of head/neck injury? (Loss of consciousness / nausea / vomiting / headache)

- Time of injury and time since last eating/drinking (relevant if going to theatre, patient will need to be starved (NBM) 6 hours before general anaesthetic)

- Visual disturbance: diplopia / loss of vision / blurred vision, visual fields. Important to check upward gaze (inferior rectus muscle entrapment)

If suspicion of head injury has not been cleared by a medical doctor, this must be undertaken prior to further maxillofacial involvement unless ABCDE indicates otherwise.

MH

- Past and current medical conditions

- Current medications (prescribed, herbal or OTC)

- Allergies, and the response to the allergen

SH

- Smoking, tobacco or other

- Alcohol, currently still intoxicated?

- Recreational drug use/addiction

- Employment and living circumstances

- If interpersonal violence cause, police involvement dependent on patient's wishes.

If the patient is unconscious, aim to gain information using the AMPLE acronym.

Allergy, Mechanism, Past medical history, Last meal, and Events before/after trauma.

Examination

Soft tissues:

- Wounds, swelling, burns, open cuts, lacerations

- Any facial asymmetry

- Blood/fluid from ears

Hard tissues:

- Any bony steps/deformity to facial skeleton

- Dental malocclusion

Visual signs

1) Loss of vision or ability to see the colour red

2) Pupils equal and reactive to light (PEARL) negative upon testing

3) Proptosis/exophthalmos – bulging eye from socket

4) Diplopia (double vision) – note if uni/bilateral and if was present prior to injury

5) Free range of eye movements (FROEM) – can the patient move their eyes in all directions without limitation or 'entrapment'

6) Subconjunctival haemorrhage – can be associated with orbital floor fractures

7) Periorbital swelling – can be palpated for surgical emphysema (cracking noises in soft tissues)

8) Bony steps in orbital rim

9) In children: do not miss a "white-eyed blowout fracture."

   ¤ Patients under 18 have slightly more elastic bones than in adults, and in trauma, the inferior rectus muscle may get trapped at the site of the orbital floor fracture. Patients may not show any clinical signs of orbital entrapment. Patients may present with nausea and vomiting for no obvious reason. Have a low threshold for a CT scan of the orbits.

For signs 1, 2 and 3, an urgent course of action is required, and a senior should be called, as the patient is showing signs of retrobulbar haemorrhage or intracranial injury.

Cranial Nerve examination

- CN V – touch sensation to three branches of the face

- CV VII – motor movements of the muscles of facial expression

Intra-oral assessment:

- Mouth opening, interincisal measurement in mm

- TMJ pain, deviation, clicks, crepitus

- Occlusion (Class I/II/III, premature contact, anterior open bite)

- Occlusal steps or gingival tears

- Sublingual haematoma (this is a fractured mandible until proven otherwise)

- Dentition: make a note of traumatised/missing/mobile teeth

- Alveolar bone/mandibular segment mobility

What special investigations would you request?

If you suspect a zygoma fracture, you will need to request

- "Facial views" X-ray facial bones – 2 occipitomental views, one at OM 30° and OM 10°

- "OPT and PA mandible" OPT and posteroanterior mandible if you suspect mandibular fracture

- These patients sometimes have a CT head to rule out any intracranial injury. It is possible to view the zygomatic complex on a standard CT head, but not below this level unless requested.

What are your differential diagnoses?

Zygomatic complex fracture signs and symptoms:

- Flattening of the cheek, asymmetry due to bony depression, often difficult to assess immediately post-injury due to soft tissue swelling.

- Numbness in the infraorbital nerve region

- Tenderness over the zygomatic arch – bony crepitus

- Infraorbital rim step

- Subconjunctival haemorrhage

- Unilateral epistaxis

- Check for trismus as this could be due to impaction of the coronoid process under the fractured arch

This could also be an orbital floor or wall fracture. Consider a CT of facial bones.

If this is a zygomatic complex fracture, how would you manage it?

1) Prompt referral for ophthalmology if you suspect any eye issues

2) If you are a DCT and you have not done a maxillofacial job before, you will need to discuss this with a senior colleague (StR on call)

3) Arrange a review in 3–5 days in an outpatient clinic to allow time for the swelling to reduce

4) Inform the patient not to blow their nose, to prevent surgical emphysema around the eye

5) Consider oral antibiotics (Co-amoxiclav 625mg TDS for 5 days)

6) Arrange an orthoptics outpatient review if the patient is experiencing any diplopia/eye signs

7) Appropriate analgesia

Consider how the patient is getting home. Ensure he is not driving, especially if you suspect any eye signs!

2 Clinical governance and risk management

What is this?

In the past, candidates were asked general questions about their achievements and research during this station. With the introduction of the portfolio station for DCT 2 and 3, this freestyle manner of questioning has reduced, and the questions are far more objective, to make it easier to mark consistently between candidates.

For DCT the questions will revolve around the principles of clinical governance and your understanding of different principles within research.

Clinical governance encompasses three main areas:

- **Culture** – educates, teaches clinicians using their mistakes, shares good practice, welcomes new practice

- **Ways of working** – to ensure patients are treated safely and appropriately with the most up to date techniques

- **Systems** – to ensure effective CPD for all members of the dental team, clinical audit, peer review, risk management.

Topics to revise are:

- The 7 pillars of Clinical Governance: CAREPUS/PACER PIRATES

- GDC Standards and CPD

- Audit and peer review

- Quality assurance: infection control, child protection, radiography guidelines, environmental safety, staff, patient and public safety

- Hierarchy of evidence

- Critical appraisal of a paper

- Definitions of audit/QUIPS/research

What is expected of you?

You will be expected to

- Define audit/QUIPS/research/service improvement

- Understand how an audit works

- Be able to provide an example of an audit you have completed

- Highlight what change in practice was made by your audit

- Address the limitations of your audit

- Be able to discuss the importance of research and how to critically appraise a paper

How long do I get?

In previous years, 3 minutes has been given beforehand to read the scenario (which will usually be face down under the chair outside of the room). You are not allowed to write notes, but should read the brief clearly and understand what the station wants you to demonstrate. Importantly, you may not be given any questions to read; it may merely be a short brief outlining what the topic of the station is. Following this, you will be asked to enter the room, where you will begin by speaking to the panel of assessors.

In previous years, 10 minutes has been allocated to this station. The assessors will usually begin by asking questions from a pre-determined list. A buzzer may be heard 1 minute before the end of the station.

How are you marked?

There will be a list of questions on a card in front of the examiner, which you will not be able to see. To score top marks, you will need to answer all the questions to a high level of accuracy to justify the examiner awarding you a top score.

Therefore, do not spend too much time on each question as they may not cut you off. Once you have answered the question, allow the examiner to ask you the next one, to avoid losing marks. If you run out of time, you will have scored zero on the unasked/unanswered questions.

The examiners are looking for your understanding of research and audit, which are integral components of a dental core training post.

Who will examine you?

You will have two examiners, who may be:

- Maxillofacial consultants

- Clinicians and consultants from a dental hospital

They may also be current educational supervisors in a secondary care setting, current postgraduate deans, and other members of the deanery.

Example of the DCT clinical governance questions

Example questions:

What is the definition of an audit?

The definition from NICE is:

"A quality improvement process that seeks to improve patient care and outcomes through systematic review of care against explicit criteria and the implementation of change"

Essentially, it is looking at the quality of patient care we are providing and seeing how we can improve it through systematic reviews. It is essential you have your own take on this and do not repeat this word for word.

What is the process of an audit?

The audit aims to evaluate whether your clinical practice is in line with best practice.

Step 1: Select a topic based on an issue you have identified. This may be a re-audit or a new topic. Decide whether this will be local or national. You may wish to explore the topic of your audit with the local department at a team meeting to validate the idea. An audit lead would need to be appointed, and the audit confirmed with the clinical lead for this department.

Step 2: Set a standard based on current 'good practice' by doing a literature search of the best available current evidence. If a standard is not already available, then it is crucial for the department to agree a local standard.

Step 3: Collect and measure current practice: surveys, data capture forms, and spreadsheets! You should aim to define a period over which to capture data on this first cycle, and a time to analyse the results. Within a larger hospital, there may be an audit lead to contact and liaise with for support.

Step 4: Analyse and reflect on the results of the first cycle. Aim to collate results and compare data to see whether the current clinical practice is meeting the required standard. If not, why is this? Identify what the causes of this are and arrange a list of recommendations for implementing before the next cycle is carried out.

Step 5: Making a change to current practice.

If, from your data, there appears to be a deficit and clinical practice is below standard, you will need to have identified why this is, and what can be done.

This could include: changing current policies or practice, providing additional training, or implementing new systems or protocol to improve compliance. Aim to agree a period of time to allow these changes to be implemented before you re-audit.

Step 6: Conduct your second cycle to close the loop by re-auditing.

Once changes have been made, you must re-audit your practice to see whether an impact has been made. Be consistent by using the same method of data collection, standard, and analysis.

Before officially beginning your audit, you may also carry out a pilot audit. This can help you assess if patients/clinicians understand your questions, if your standards need modification, and if your data capture sheet contains all the relevant data.

Give an example of an audit you have carried out.

Common audit topics in dentistry are:

- Radiography

- Antibiotic prescribing

- BPE screening

- Record keeping

- ID block

Aim to describe how you came to identify the topic, your objectives and the methods (as described above). Focus on the change you made and whether these impacted on the clinical practice and quality of care of your patients.

What were the limitations of your audit?

Some areas to consider:

- Sample size

- Audits are mainly retrospective

- In large institutions, there may be resistance to the change implemented

- Engagement of clinicians: staffing turnover

- Skills and training of participants

- One of the biggest weaknesses within any audit cycle is not being able to 'close the audit loop/complete the audit cycle' link:

"How-to guide" on clinical audit http://www.dvh.nhs.uk/EasyS-iteWeb/GatewayLink.aspx?alId=107264

What is the strongest type of evidence?

It is important to appreciate that scientific evidence can be classified into a hierarchy of evidence (Figure 1).

In your answer, you should aim to:

- Describe this hierarchy, explaining that systematic review of randomised controlled trials is the strongest level of evidence, and the weakest is that of expert opinion

- Explain that not all evidence is equal in value

- Explain how each of the evidence levels varies (as described below)

- Describe that within each study design, it is the methodology used to minimise the bias that is the determinant of the quality of evidence

The Oxford (UK) CEBM Levels of Evidence 2009 have divided the levels of evidence in the following fashion:

Figure 1. Hierarchy of evidence

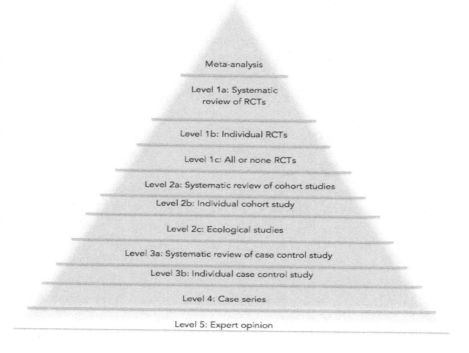

Case series and case reports: These are collections of reports that discuss an individual patient case and how they were treated. They do not use any control groups. Therefore, they have little statistical validity.

Cross-sectional study: This is an observational study that analyses data collected from an entire population at a specific moment in time.

Case-control studies: These are studies that look at patients who already have a specific condition in comparison with patients that don't.

Retrospective cohort study: This is a longitudinal study which looks at a group of individuals that share a common exposure factor to determine whether this is linked to a disease they developed in comparison with a group of individuals without this factor exposure.

Prospective cohort study: This is a type of observational study where two or more cohorts (groups) are monitored. One group has a particular risk factor or disease, and the other group does not; both groups are tracked to discover if trends occur over time.

Randomised control trial: This is a quantitative study where participants of similar characteristics (age, health, ethnicity) are allocated into random groups, one of which is a control group and the other an experimental group. The participants within the control may receive a placebo or no intervention at all, whilst the experimental group will receive the intervention being investigated. The results are statistically analysed to reduce bias.

Systematic review: This is the highest level of available evidence. Systematic reviews aim to present a summary of evidence from multiple primary studies using explicit, reproducible methods and critically appraising the evidence.

Meta-analysis: This is a statistical method used in certain systematic reviews to provide a summary result or outcome. A meta-analysis combines data from similar primary studies and integrates the findings by using reproducible statistical techniques to extract and collate data.

Therefore, not all systematic reviews use meta-analysis; only those which are reviewing studies which are of a similar nature to provide meaningful results.

Useful links:

NICE glossary: https://www.nice.org.uk/glossary

Cochrane: http://consum ers.cochrane.org/

What is evidence-based dentistry (EBD)?

Evidence-based dentistry involves decision-making using the integration of best available evidence related to the clinical situation combined with clinical expertise and knowledge and the patient's values and beliefs.

You should avoid regurgitating this definition and aim to apply your own variant of this answer. It will be useful to give an example of how you may have applied this in your practice.

This may include:

- When a patient has read something in the press regarding the detriments of a particular drug or treatment, i.e., fluoride, and you have used EBD to explain your perspective.

- When there is a particularly difficult clinical situation, and you have used EBD to help a patient make an informed decision.

Adapted from David Sackett et al. Evidence-Based Medicine: How to Practice and Teach EBM (New York: Churchill Livingstone, 2000)

3 Clinical communication

What is this?

The clinical communication station is an OSCE-type scenario, which involves you discussing the management of a patient-related clinical situation. In 2018, there were 10 minutes allocated to this station. The clinical scenario presented will mimic that of a dilemma faced by a DCT. Therefore, you will be assessed on your personal skills and professional integrity. It is important to note that this station is an assessment based mainly on your communication skills, how you interact with the patient, and your overall ability to cope with the situation. For this, you will be speaking to an actor who is the 'patient' and assessors observe you. Technical knowledge and a high level of academic theory are not assessed in this station.

How long do I get?

n the 2018 round, 3 minutes were given beforehand to read the scenario (this was face down under the chair outside of the room). You are not allowed to write notes but should read the script clearly and understand what it is that the question is asking of you. Following this, you will be asked to enter the room, where you will begin by speaking to the patient (actor). You have 10 minutes within the station; you should aim to answer the patient's principal concerns and ensure that these are managed before the time ends. You will hear a buzzer 1 minute before the end of the station.

What is expected of you?

You are expected to act as a competent, safe, and compassionate DCT.

You are expected to formulate a pragmatic and logical management plan, which will be communicated to the patient in the form of a consultation. Both the actor (patient) and the assessors will be observing your capacity to demonstrate strong interpersonal skills, planning, and the values of a DCT.

How are you marked?

There are usually two assessors, who may be consultants or experienced clinicians from a Dental Teaching Hospital. They may also be current educational supervisors in a secondary care setting, current postgraduate deans and other members of the deanery.

The assessors often remain silent and only observe your interaction with the patient. They will be busy listening to your answers and scoring you, so it is important this does not distract you when you are speaking to your patient. Assessors will be listening to your answers to award a score.

Key factors that they will be looking for:

- Successful communication with the patient, with behaviour, body language, tone and words suited to the situation and the patient

- Consideration for the patient's feelings and anxiety, with strong focus on the ability to empathise and deal with issues sensitive to the patient

- Ability to think conceptually with a holistic approach, taking into consideration the patient's beliefs, values, and wishes when considering management

- Efficient use of the team in caring for the patient, adopting a team approach, and promoting each individual's skill set

- Ability to utilise clinical time efficiently, ensure valuable use of resources, and prioritise tasks

- Demonstrating values commensurate with those of NHS values, including commitment to quality of care, respect, and dignity, compassion, working together for patients, everyone counts and improving lives.

Example of the DCT clinical communication scenario:
Undiagnosed periodontitis

Scenario 1

You have 3 minutes to read this scenario.

A 45-year-old female patient, Mrs Smith, who is a patient of your principal Dr Jones, has been booked to see you due to pain from a lower left back tooth.

The patient has been complaining that this tooth has become increasingly loose, and the patient is concerned.

C/O: Wobbly and painful lower back tooth

RMH: Atorvastatin, Bisoprolol

SH: 20 cigarettes per day, nil alcohol

Frequent dental attendance to see the principal

Nil interdental cleaning but use of electric toothbrush

Mildly anxious

Today:

You have taken an OPG radiograph and have conducted a full clinical examination. There are no systemic signs or symptoms.

Findings:

E/O: NAD

I/O : STE: Bilateral linea alba on buccal mucosa along occlusal plane.

BPE:

4	4	4
4	4	4

Gingivae: Red, inflamed, loss of contour. Halitosis

Hard tissues:

All maxillary teeth non-mobile, LL7 is grade 3 mobile, TTP and a deep PPD is found on the mesial surface with bleeding.

OPT radiograph (present in the room) showing:

- 90% bone loss around LL7 with furcation involvement

- Up to 30% horizontal bone loss in maxilla and 40 % horizontal loss in mandible

- No coronal radiolucencies or other abnormalities.

Questions

1) **Explain to the patient the findings and your management**

2) **Explain why the tooth is painful**

3) **Questions you are *likely* to be asked by patient: Why hasn't this been identified earlier? What is going to be done about the tooth? When can this be done? Will I lose my other teeth? How can this be resolved?**

Typical answer

Italics = Suggested dialogue

Context

The scenario is usually placed face down on the floor, beneath a chair, outside of the room you will be assessed within. You will have 3 minutes to read through this and prepare a mental answer (there is no paper or pen allowed).

Following the timed 3 minutes of reading, you would be expected to enter the room and begin.

Answer structure

You will have 10 minutes to speak with the patient (actor), who will be interacting with you throughout and asking questions.

- Acknowledge the patient with a greeting, such as *'Hello, my name is Dr (Name), I am a colleague of Dr Jones. I work here at the practice.'*

- Two-factor identification – check address and DOB *'Just to make sure we have the correct notes, please can I confirm your details…'*

- Show empathy: *'I am so sorry to hear about your toothache. We will take all the steps we need to resolve this for you today.'*

Explaining the findings

Be creative and improvise

- (Holding a piece of paper provided with the scenario) *'Here we can see your x-ray, this shows the top teeth, and we can see your bone levels on the bottom jaw have shrunk back.'*

- Give a jargon-free answer (avoid using terminology such as periodontal condition, sub-gingival calculus or root surface debridement. Use patient-friendly phrases, such as: bacteria growing around the gum margin, deep cleanse of the gum and root surface, hardened bacterial growing along the tooth and gum.

- Give a clear explanation of the process without confusing the patient.

- Stop to ask, chunk and check information; provide a short amount of information and reconfirm with the patient that they are clear about what you have told them.

- Ask patients questions that allow you to lead them to an answer *'Have you heard of gum disease before, Mrs Smith? ... Would you like me to explain this to you?'*

- Explaining dental pathology in a way that the patient (actor) understands is paramount, as once they understand this, they can relate to how management will help them.

- Use of visual aids to assist patients can work well such as using a pen to describe a tooth and the hand as the bone around it. As you lose bone through periodontitis, the hand (representing the bone) moves further down the pen, so the tooth (pen) is less well supported; this can be directly shown to the patient and works very well.

TIP: The actor will also score you during these scenarios, so it is essential you impress them and build a good rapport.

Management

The patient wants to know how this is going to be resolved and due to being in such pain wants this done today.

Immediate management

- Explain the cause of the patient's pain, identify which tooth is symptomatic, and manage this, considering the patient's overall dental health condition and acute pain.

- *'It shows from looking in the mouth today and your x-rays that the lower back molar tooth has a large infection around the root surface where bacteria has built up causing an abscess, in addition to widespread periodontitis, or gum disease'*

Plan should include:

A) Methods of treatment possible for the symptomatic LL7 tooth:

1. Relief of pain – knowing the tooth is grade III mobile, it is prudent to extract, offering various modalities of treatment (LA, LA+Sedation or potentially a general anaesthetic referral) – aim to explain the advantages, disadvantages, risks, and benefits of treatment.

Advantages include: Relief of pain, removal of infection, and prevention of aspirating or swallowing the loose tooth.

Disadvantages include: Loss of a functional tooth, pain following the treatment, bleeding, bruising, swelling, risk of infection, jaw ache and dry socket (early loss of blood clot or failure to form).

2. The option of no treatment should be offered but advising patient the risks of this, i.e. further pain, increasing size of infection, risk of aspiration or eventual loss of tooth.

For the remaining dentition, you must create a plan, and discussion should include:

1) (A detailed oral hygiene visit and help to stop smoking) Oral hygiene appointment, smoking cessation advice.

2) (A deep clean) Full 6PPD charting and RSD (deep clean with LA if needed).

3) (A follow-up and additional clean appointment) Review of the gum health with the hygienist.

This should be phrased without jargon!

- *'We know that certain triggers are likely to increase your risk of gum disease. These include smoking and bacteria around the gum margin. Some people have a much stronger reaction to bacteria, and their gum disease progresses faster. Whilst we cannot cure this, we can certainly control and prevent it from worsening. Would you like that?'*

- *'In order to restore your gums to a healthy state, I would strongly advise you visit our hygiene team who will help develop a personalised care plan for your gums and teeth, starting with removing the factors that can increase tooth loss, such as bacteria around the gums and smoking.'*

- *'You will likely then need to return for a deeper clean to remove bacteria stuck to the root surface. This will help improve your gum health and make your teeth firmer; we can also use a numbing injection, so you are comfortable throughout. Are you happy with this, Mrs Smith?'*

- Explain that therapy can begin as soon as possible and this will help to prolong the life of the remaining teeth and help prevent the condition from worsening.

- Explain the risk factors associated with periodontitis, including smoking, poor OH, and plaque control, and relate these directly to the patient.

The patient is frustrated that this was not identified sooner and requests a reason why this has only been detected now.

A good candidate will:

- Acknowledge the patient's frustration and dismay. Remember that non-verbal behaviour comprises 93% of communication (55% body language, 38% tone) and the remaining 7% is verbal.

- Apologise to the patient that she is in discomfort and that these are symptoms of her condition; reassure her that the condition is not sinister but can result in pain and mobile teeth.

- Apologise also that it is you that has to inform her of the news and not the principal.

- Advise and reassure the patient that whilst this is the case, you will ensure that a reason is sought from the principal as to why they have not informed the patient and that she will receive an explanation.

- Offer the patient a resolution – advising that although she has come in with pain today, you can relieve this and develop a personal oral health plan to prevent the disease from getting worse.

- Only if the patient expresses a desire to make a complaint should you begin to offer the patient a complaints leaflet and inform them about the process, as ideally, you wish to resolve this locally and avoid escalating the situation.

Towards the end of the 10 minutes, you will hear a 1-r warning.

In this period, you should do three things:

1) Summarise by explaining your findings and the management plan with the patient.

2) Provide the patient with an opportunity to ask any questions.

3) Provide the patient with your name and contact details, patient information leaflet, and information where they can research more about the condition, such as the Oral Health Foundation website and independent hotline.

Remember this is an actor, so communication is vital. Practise on patients and family members who have no dental background. If you are able to master discussing difficult cases with them, you will be in a strong position to discuss scenarios with actors.

The Situational Judgment Test

For the 2019 DCT recruitment process, the SJT will be conducted on a separate date to the selection centre interview, at a Pearson VUE test centre.

You will be sent an invitation via Oriel for the SJT on Monday 11th March 2019 at 6pm, and the SJT assessments will occur between Wednesday 20th March and Wednesday 27th 2019.

Subsequently, selection centre invitations will be sent to applicants on Tuesday 2nd April 2019 at 6pm, with a deadline for selecting interview slots on Friday 5th April 2019 at 6pm. The selection centre assessment occurs between Monday 29th April 2019 and Friday 3rd May 2019.

What is the SJT?

For DCT 1 applicants, the Situational Judgment Test is a formal examination, which accounts for 25% of the overall applicant score (with the remaining 75% made from the clinical communication, clinical scenario, and clinical governance and risk management stations, at a weighting of 25% each).

For DCT 2 and 3 applicants the SJT accounts for 20% of the overall applicant score, with the remaining 80% divided among the clinical communication, clinical scenario, and clinical governance and risk management stations.

The SJT is a method of assessing your professional and personal attributes and is a non-academic test. Written with the help of psychologists and clinicians and approved by a consensus panel of dentistry specialists and consultants, the SJT contains clinical dilemmas which may be encountered by DCTs. The SJT ultimately aims to test an applicant's probity, decision-making, professionalism, and ability to manage pressurised situations.

The SJT assessment is conducted in formal examination conditions and in 2018 lasted 115 minutes (1 hour 55 minutes). The SJT contained questions with multi-choice answers.

These SJT questions were formatted into two categories of questions including ranking and best three answers. Ranking questions involve reading a short passage of text, which often involves a clinical dilemma or ethical issue, and then ranking the pre-determined answers from 1 to 5 based on what should be done, as a DCT, in the clinical context of the question. The best three answers questions involve selecting the three best answers available, from eight pre-determined answers.

2019 is the second year the DCT SJT assessment will be conducted on a computer at a Pearson VUE test centre. To ensure you are completely aware of the new process, you are advised to read the COPDEND applicants' guide, available on the COP-DEND website, which will detail the process by which the SJT will be undertaken.

Improving your score

Practise, learn and test

Practice does not make perfect, it makes permanent. It is, therefore, important that you learn the specific technique of how to answer the SJT questions.

It is certain that preparation for the SJT cannot be crammed in. You will need to spend time developing the correct technique by understanding and answering the questions, before progressing onto timed mock questions. The SJT requires regular practice to understand how the answers are justified, and mock tests under timed, exam conditions, to best prepare you for the day.

Rank worst and best first

Unfortunately, it is difficult to create a set of rules to apply to each and every dilemma. However, as a guide to saving you time, aim to answer the first and fifth preferences first. By answering the first and fifth choices initially, you will clear two options quickly, and have the potential to gain most marks (they also have the potential to lose most marks if ranked incorrectly), so it is important to establish these first.

Read twice, answer once

Although you have a limited amount of time per question, it is more important to read the question thoroughly than to rush to answer it. Although it is important to complete as many questions as possible, reading the question and understanding the dilemma is key to choosing your preferred answers.

Sorting middle options

Regarding ranking questions, once you have selected the first and fifth choice preferences, you must aim to distinguish between the remaining three options.

Generally, those answers that tend to be lower down the preference include actions that compromise patient safety, behaviour that is unprofessional, or decisions that may lead to worsening of the situation such as violence, negative morale, or a complaint.

Answers that may be considered highly preferred include actions that promote patient safety, quality of care and clinical efficiency, behaviour that shows respect and dignity for patients and staff, or actions that demonstrate good teamwork, initiative and acting within your limitations.

Act as a DCT

In each scenario, the most appropriate thing to do is to act within your own limits, as patient safety is key. Remember that it is an assessment of your personal attributes, so answering as a responsible and safe DCT is paramount.

Answers that allow you to seek help from a senior colleague or trainer should be preferred to taking on too much responsibility and threatening patient safety.

Don't overthink

Remember that you have a limited time per question. In this time, it is essential to have read and understood the question and left sufficient time to make an informed judgment on the remaining answers.

It is important to note that within the SJT there are no negative marks, and points are awarded for 'near misses'; therefore, you should aim to complete all questions for a maximum chance of scoring highly.

How will I be assessed?

For each ranking question, a maximum of 20 points can be awarded, with the lowest score being 8 points. For each correctly ranked answer, 4 points are awarded; points will be deducted for each incorrect answer, with more points lost the further away from the correct answer you are. Therefore it is possible to lose 8 points if you were to get the first and last preference mixed up.

For example, if the correct ranking order for a particular question is EDCBA, and you rank every answer correctly, you will score 20 points. However, if you answer this as ABCDE, you will score 8 points only (Table 3).

Table 3. How the ranking SJT score is determined

Correct rank	Applicant rank 1st	Applicant rank 2nd	Applicant rank 3rd	Applicant rank 4th	Applicant rank 5th
	A	B	C	D	E
E	4	3	2	1	0
D	3	4	3	2	1
C	2	3	4	3	2
B	1	2	3	4	3
A	0	1	2	3	4
Score =8					

Best three answers

You will have eight pre-determined answers to choose from within this category of questions. You must only select the three most appropriate options that work synergistically to answer the question.

It is, therefore, important to first discount all options that do not seem sensible, to leave three to five remaining answers. From then it is important to follow the principles discussed above, but ensure that the three options do not contradict one another. The answers chosen should reflect the response of a diligent DCT.

For each correct answer, there are 4 points awarded, so you can score a maximum of 12 points per question or a minimum of 0.

Your overall rank

Based on your performance at the assessment stations and the SJT, you will be assigned a national ranking: a score ranging from number one to the total number of interviewed applicants. This is called a Single Transferrable Score (STS) and allows you to be allocated to posts across the UK and not just the region of your selection centre.

In order to be considered 'appointable,' you must score at least 40% across the three stations at the selection centre. If your scores do not reach the appointable thresholds, then you will not be considered for recruitment, and a post will not be offered to you.

Appointment of posts

Offers are made in rank order and will be based on the highest-preferred post when your rank is reached. Therefore, if you ranked the position of DCT 1 OMFS in Queen Elizabeth

Hospital West Midlands as your first choice, and were the highest-ranking candidate that preferenced this post, this would be offered to you first. The next candidate who ranked this as their first choice and was the second-highest ranking candidate would be offered the position next, and so on until the post fills up. First-choice post holders cannot upgrade or downgrade, but may accept or reject the offers.

If, however you ranked this post as your first choice, but the two positions for this role had been accepted and you happened to be the third-highest ranked candidate, you would not be offered this. You would, however, be able to accept a post elsewhere with upgrades. This means that if any of the applicants who were offered your preferred post decide to decline it, and spaces become available, then this post will become available to you.

It is important to note that if posts are declined or are not accepted on time, you will be left without a job; therefore, be very aware of the Oriel deadlines.

Chapter 3

Mock Scenarios

Clinical Scenario

Example 1

You are an OMFS DCT working in a busy emergency department. A 14-year-old child attends in pain with her uncle. You go out to the waiting room to call her in and notice the uncle is on the phone and indicates to you to carry out the assessment whilst he finishes his call.

The child has limited English and appears quite withdrawn and nervous. You understand that she is in significant pain arising from her lower left first molar.

Upon assessment, you notice she has several grossly carious teeth and the following BPE scores

BPE:

3	2	3
2	2	3

You go out to the waiting room to ask the uncle to come in, but he is asleep and smells of alcohol. Other patients have informed the receptionist about his erratic and rowdy behaviour. Once you have woken him, he enters the surgery, and you explain your findings to him. You suspect he is not translating the information to her accurately.

Questions they may ask:

What are the main issues here?

The main issues are patient safety, child safeguarding, and consent.

The patient has attended an appointment for her pain. You have noticed a state of poor overall dental health. The patient may have no oral hygiene regimen, and this will need to be addressed along with her other dental problems to ensure the problems do not progress. It is important that follow-up appointments are made to carry out treatment.

The patient is a 14-year-old girl, therefore legally a child. She can give consent as long as she is able to be deemed competent. It is mentioned in the scenario that the patient has a limited understanding of English. The level of understanding needs to be gauged as the patient may be able to consent for treatment on an emergency basis, with further, more complex treatment explained with the help of an interpreter.

The girl has attended the appointment with her uncle, who you suspect is under the influence of alcohol. Suspicions may be raised when the uncle who brought her to the appointment is not correctly translating the information. Further investigation as to the relationship of the uncle to the patient is warranted, as well as the location of the patient's parents, and if they are able to consent for treatment for the patient if they have a better understanding of English, or are able to translate accurately for consent.

How would you manage this scenario?

- Attempt to contact the patient's parents to inform them of the treatment plan and to gain their consent.

- Effectively treat the patient for her pain following gaining consent from the patient.

- If you have any suspicion regarding the quality of the translation ask LanguageLine to translate over the phone.

- If there is any suspicion that the patient is being coerced, ask the uncle to leave the room. Ensure a chaperone is present at all times.

- Book the patient in for further appointments.

- If you have any concerns regarding the patient's safety, contact the local safeguarding team to inform them.

You explain the importance of addressing the pain and infection in her mouth, but the uncle is very dismissive and begins to leave the surgery with the girl, pulling her by her arm from the dental chair. He tells you that she does not need to have treatment.

How do you respond?

- It is important to maintain professionalism and act in a non-confrontational manner, so as not to escalate the situation with a member of the public who you suspect is under the influence of alcohol.

- The uncle cannot refuse dental treatment unless he has been deemed to be the legal guardian of the child.

If you suspect that by grabbing the patient by the arm there is a physical form of abuse occurring, contact the police and inform the child-safeguarding team for the local area.

What could you do in the long term?

- Notify the local area team.

- Try to contact the patient on the contact details provided to attend for a further appointment with a view to keeping a close eye on her social situation.

Example 2

It is 3pm., and you are the OMFS DCT on call for a large tertiary centre. You receive a phone call from a local dentist. She explains that she has carried out an extraction of the LR7 on her patient, Mr Williams, this morning and the patient has returned with a bleeding socket. The bleeding has not stopped since he left the surgery at 10am.

What are the questions you need to ask the dentist before taking the referral?

- Further patient details: age and medical history of the patient; is the patient on any anticoagulant medications/clotting disorders?

- Nature of the extraction: surgical, simple, carious tooth, abscess associated, any retained roots

- Nature of the post-operative bleeding: slow ooze or rapidly flowing bright red (arterial) blood

- Has the patient attempted local measures at home, e.g. haemostasis with pressure?

- Has the dentist attempted any local measures, e.g. packing/suturing?

What advice can you give the dentist on the phone?

- Isolate where the bleeding is coming from, use aspiration to ascertain if bleeding is active, coming from bone or gingiva

- Local measures such as haemostatic agents (haemocollagen/surgicel)

- Gauze soaked in dental local anaesthetic (LA) with adrenaline

- Local infiltration of LA with adrenaline

- Suturing of bleeding gingiva under tension

You discover in the medical history that the patient has a Factor VIII deficiency, and you decide to take this referral. When the patient arrives, what is your initial management?

- ABCDE approach

- Thorough history from the patient

- Check vital signs for hypovolaemic shock (low blood pressure, high heart rate)

- Examine the patient and assess bleed

- Take bloods if patient looks unwell/severe bleed: FBC, U+E, LFT, Clotting screen, Group and Save

Which other teams may you need to liaise with?

- Haematology team and A&E senior if massive blood loss. (Inform them you are only dentally qualified.)

- The patient with haemophilia A will most likely be known to them.

- They will know the extent of the coagulopathy and the best course of management.

What could you prescribe in a hospital setting?

- Tranexamic acid PO (oral) or M/W (mouthwash)

How might you prevent this for future extractions for this patient?

- Consider referral to OMFS for dental extractions under LA.

- Liaison with haematology can be undertaken before extraction.

- Systemic desmopressin or Factor VIII can be given IV before extraction to boost the patient's coagulation.

Example 3

You are a DCT in a maxillofacial unit looking after the oncology patients on the ward. One of your patients, Helen, underwent major surgery 10 days ago: she had a surgical resection of an SCC from the left side of her tongue, tracheostomy, bilateral neck dissection and reconstruction with a radial forearm free flap. You notice she appears to look quite unwell today, and the nurses alert you to a rise in her temperature, which is now 38.4 degrees.

You go to assess the patient. What other signs do you look for?

Patient observations include:

- Temperature

- Heart rate (pulse)

- Blood pressure

- Respiratory rate

- Oxygen saturation

- Urine output

Case-specific

- Free flap: Colour, capillary refill time, warmth of the skin flap, texture of skin flap.

- Tracheostomy secretions – assess if there is mucus/blood being coughed up from the tracheostomy site and the nature of these secretions.

- Drains from the surgical site – these would have been placed intra-operatively and allow for excess fluid to be drained whilst the swelling settles and prevent collection of fluid.

What are you concerned about?

- Infection – this can be from the surgical site or from a chest infection as a result of being immobile for a number of days following surgery.

- Flap failure – if the skin flap looks mottled or dusky grey/blue, sluggish or very fast capillary refill time, is cold or splitting away (dehiscence) from the body, call your OMFS senior immediately.

- Post-operative bleeding – the patient has had some reconnection of blood vessels; should a vessel rupture, the patient will lose a large amount of blood quickly.

- Compartment syndrome: if tissue has been taken from another site of the body (leg or forearm) there is a chance there can be a bleed within the forearm or leg. This can be seen by assessing the limb for the 6 P's: *Pain, pale* limb, *pulseless, paraesthesia, paralysis, perishingly* cold limb – call your OMFS senior.

How might you manage this?

- Look at other observations to see if any other factors are leading to a diagnosis.

- Inform a senior member of the OMFS team such as the Registrar or Consultant, and take advice on how to proceed.

- Ensure there is a patent cannula to allow administration of fluids and antibiotics if required.

- Inform the nurse looking after the patient to keep a close eye on what you are concerned about.

- Document your findings accurately in the notes.

Example 4

You are the maxillofacial DCT on call. A 27-year-old woman attends with a large swelling arising from what you suspect is a tooth abscess. You are concerned as she has got a raised temperature and worsening trismus.

How would you assess this patient?

ABCDE

Risk of losing airway by the spread of abscess around airway/trismus:

Signs of airway obstruction are:

- Bilateral raised floor of mouth

- Drooling

- Difficulty swallowing

- Husky voice (hot potato voice)

- Patient sitting up forward; cannot lie flat.

Other factors indicating a large swelling which may be an emergency include:

- Pyrexia

- Restricted mouth opening (trismus)

- Swelling crossing the midline

- Rapidly progressing swelling (take thorough history if possible)

- Increased white blood cell and CRP levels on blood count

What investigations would you need to carry out?

- OPG to determine which tooth may be the cause of the dental abscess

- Full blood count, urea, and electrolytes, c-reactive protein (CRP), lactate, liver function tests (LFTs), group and save (most likely going to need to operate)

- CT of the head and neck is sometimes done to determine if there is a collection of pus which can be drained – (discuss this with your senior)

How might you manage this patient immediately?

- Take a full history of the swelling, how quickly it came on, any antibiotics that have been prescribed previously.

- Note when the patient last ate or drank anything.

- Cannulate to provide systemic antibiotics and fluid.

- Ensure all radiographs are available. If there is a local collection intraorally, carry out incision and drainage of the abscess under local anaesthetic.

- Inform a senior member of staff and seek a second opinion should you be in any doubt.

You suspect the swelling extends into the buccal space, and it is not something you will be able to drain locally. What is your management plan and who might you involve?

- Admit the patient, cannulate the patient, taking baseline bloods, and begin fluids if needed.

- Place the patient on the emergency list; this will involve informing the emergency coordinator and providing details of how urgent the procedure is.

- Inform the first on-call anaesthetist of the patient's details, diagnosis, trismus, medical history, and blood results. The patient will need to be placed under a general anaesthetic (due to the limited mouth opening and the operating site being intraoral, the anaesthetist may have to place the tube through the nose). Inform the anaesthetist of how urgent the operation is – discuss with your senior to grade this.

Clinical governance and risk management

Why do you think research is important in dentistry?

There are two factors to consider in your answer:

- The impact on the practice/trust/hospital/department

- The importance to you as a training dentist

The institute you work within may gain national or international recognition for the research and, therefore, can improve its reputation. This may lead to better patient outcomes through improved practice, a higher calibre of staff, and further funding. Also, successful clinical trials may allow patients within that hospital or department to gain first use of novel therapy or treatments.

For you as a training dentist, understanding research and the hierarchy of evidence will allow you to understand and differentiate between good and poor quality evidence. When used in clinical decisions, and taking into account patient values, this will enable you to make informed, evidence-based decisions.

Research is also essential as dentistry is continually developing; therefore, keeping up to date with current relevant high-quality evidence ensures that patients are given the best available treatments to improve outcomes.

Undertaking research also allows training dentists to experience the academic pathway of dentistry and may encourage dentists to become involved with research projects or trials aiming to help further innovation and improve dental health.

What clinical governance activities have you undertaken?

Clinical governance is a process of ensuring high standards of care are maintained, through the NHS taking accountability to its patients.

Traditionally, clinical governance has been described with 7 pillars:

- *Clinical effectiveness and research*

- *Audit*

- *Risk management*

- *Education and training*

- Patient and public involvement

- Using information and IT

- Staffing and staff management

The first four pillars (CARE) are more related to the DCT. You should begin by explaining, in your own words, your understanding of these and give examples of how you have involved these aspects of clinical governance within your practice.

Clinical effectiveness and research examples include using evidence-based dentistry to manage patients that you treat, or conducting or being involved with research that aims to improve the care of patients.

Audit examples are mentioned in the previous chapter (Chapter 2). Aim to detail how your audit made a change and how this change led to improved patient care.

Risk management is described below.

Education and training involve regularly updating knowledge. You should show how you are a self-directed learner and describe how the CPD courses and conferences you have attended have improved your knowledge and skills to improve your clinical practice. You can also evidence your training through completing an online portfolio, such as the DFT portfolio, where you can show your observed clinical procedures and workplace assessments.

What is risk management?

Risk management is an element of clinical governance that entails the processes of understanding, identifying and minimising risks to patients and staff.

Risk, in the context of the dental setting, is any uncertainty of outcome that may occur during clinical care or treatment that may have an adverse effect on patients or staff. An important aspect of strengthening risk management protocol involves an open, blame-free culture, and an environment where mistakes and experiences can be shared for the benefit of everyone.

The classic risk management cycle involves four stages:

1) Identifying the risks by understanding what and how adverse outcomes may arise during clinical care.

2) Analysing the risk – what are the chances of this occurring, and what is the outcome of the risk and the consequence to the patient and staff?

3) Controlling the risk – how can the chances of this risk be minimised?

4) Transferring the risk – are you able to refer patients to minimise risk?

When identifying why an adverse outcome has happened, the use of root cause analysis tools such as the Ishikawa cause and effect 'fishbone' diagram or the 'five whys' questions may help give further information constructively.

What is an audit spiral?

This is when you are due to conduct a re-audit (second cycle) to close the audit loop; however, in the period between the first and second cycle, there has been a change in the standard, i.e. the level of care expected has changed. Therefore, this will require you to conduct a new audit, and this is considered an 'audit spiral'.

What is the difference between audit and research?

You must be able to clearly differentiate between research and audit.

With an audit, you are assessing current practice in line with best practice using a set standard, whilst research aims to find out whether new treatments or therapies work and their clinical effectiveness. Therefore, with an audit, you are establishing whether best practice is being used, but with research you are finding out what the best practice is.

Other key differences include:

- Audits measure compliance with set standards in accordance with guidelines, whilst research aims to discover new information and uses null and alternative hypotheses.

- Audits do not involve allocation of participants into random groups.

- Audits do not involve experimental interventions, whilst research may do.

- Research requires ethical approval, whilst audits rarely do.

What are the GDC CPD requirements for dentists?

From 1st January 2018, dentist shave been on the enhanced CPD scheme set out by the GDC. Dentists are required to complete 100 hours of verifiable CPD in a five-year cycle. It must be spaced out to ensure there are 10 hours of verifiable CPD during any 2-year period.

The three core CPD topics are:

1) Medical Emergencies: 10 hours in every CPD cycle (at least 2 hours of medical emergency CPD every 2 years)

2) Disinfection and decontamination: At least 5 hours in each CPD cycle

3) Radiography and radiation protection: At least 5 hours in every CPD cycle

Other GDC-recommended CPD topics are:

- Legal and ethical issues

- Complaints handling

- Oral cancer: early detection

- Vulnerable adult safeguarding

- Safeguarding of children and young adults

You should know how many hours are required for each core CPD topic and also the requirements for Dental Care Professionals.

Clinical Communication

You have 3 minutes to read this scenario.

<u>Example 1</u>

You are a DCT in an Oral Medicine unit at a Dental Teaching Hospital. You have been referred a 56-year-old man from a local practice who has presented with a suspicious white and red patch on the lateral border of his tongue. The referral letter states that he has had this patch for 2 months and although it is not causing him any pain, it is getting bigger and therefore he was referred to you via the two-week pathway. You note the following information on the letter:

RMH: Patient takes warfarin and had a stroke in 2016.

SH: He has smoked 20 cigarettes a day for 40 years and consumes 20 units of alcohol per week. The patient works as a bricklayer.

DH: Brushes 1x day. Does not attend the dentist regularly. Dentally anxious.

Question:

The patient is here to see you today for a consultation, and you will need to advise him that this lesion will require a biopsy.

Answer:

The actor is very nervous during this scenario, especially over having a local anaesthetic. He is also very worried that he has cancer.

Introduction and rapport building

- Greet the patient in an open and friendly manner.

- Introduce yourself and advise him how you are going to help.

- Check patient name, address, and date of birth.

- Establish why the patient has attended today and confirm their understanding. *'I understand you have been referred here by your dentist, due to a red and white area on your tongue — is this correct, sir?'*

- Collect a short history. *'I understand that this has been here for 2 months. Is it painful? Has it grown in size? Have you had similar areas like this before?'*

- Check medical health and any medications or allergies – although it is stated in the referral letter, you have not personally seen this patient yourself previously, and therefore you must ask. You could simply ask *'other than the stroke you had in 2016, do you have any other medical conditions? Are you taking anything other than warfarin?'*

- Check smoking and alcohol status (if you suspect other habits, it may be prudent to ask about chewing tobacco, betel nut or paan).

- Ask about employment status and availability for appointments.

Explain your management

- *'So I've had a look at the area, and it appears to be a mixed patch on the side of your tongue. We can't quite confirm what it is by looking at it, so we'll need to do a biopsy, which means we'll need to take a sample of it.'*

- It may be worth asking if the patient has had a biopsy before.

You note that the patient is very anxious and resistant about proceeding with the biopsy.

Address the patient's concerns

- Patient anxiety: Aim to seek why it is that the patient is worried.

- Anxiety management: Reassure, empathise, and provide the patient with options to manage this. For example, if he is needle phobic, intravenous sedation may not be the best option, as it will still require a needle. However, inhalation sedation may work well with the use of topical anaesthetic.

- Find out what he is nervous about; ask specifically, e.g., LA used for dental treatment, needles in general or the sound of the drill, etc.

- *'It's quite a simple procedure and will involve taking a small sample of the cells from that area for our laboratory* to examine them under a microscope so we can give you a diagnosis as to what this might be.'

- The actor may ask specific questions about why he is having the biopsy done.

Typical questions may include:

'Do I have cancer?'

- 'We can't quite tell looking at it what this might be. It could be a lot of things, but we wouldn't be able to know without testing the cells in that area.'

'What does the procedure involve?'

- 'It will involve giving you some local anaesthetic which will numb your tongue up on that side so that you don't feel anything.'

- 'We will then take a small sample of the area and put in some dissolvable stitches to close it afterwards.'

- 'It may ooze a little throughout the day afterwards, but we will give you all the post-op care after the procedure and tell you how to look after it.'

Obtain consent

- There will be a set number of marks available for risks and benefits of the procedure and how you explain these to patients.

- 'Today we will be getting your consent for sampling (biopsy) of the tissue from the side of your left tongue. Is that right?'

- The benefits of the procedure are to aid diagnosis and help treat the patient appropriately.

- As the patient is on warfarin, in accordance with the SDCEP guidelines, it is important to inform the patient that an INR test will be done before so that haemostasis can be managed (this may be done on site with a portable INR machine). It is worth mentioning that due to this medication there can be an increased risk of bleeding after treatment.

- The risks of the procedure are: Bleeding, swelling, bruising, post-op infection (which is a higher risk in smokers), post-op pain (which can be managed with over-the-counter painkillers), sutures, failure to diagnose meaning a second procedure may be required. Depending on location, you may need to warn for paraesthesia and anaesthesia, i.e., lower lip region.

After further probing, you realise the patient is worried as he cannot get time off work – a good candidate will take into consideration their work commitments and tailor the appointment to them.

Follow up and aftercare

- Reassure the patient that you can book appointments around them and aim to schedule an appointment date today so they know when they can take time off for the biopsy.

- Print an appointment card so they do not forget and advise them you can call them prior to the day to check they can still make it.

- Advise them that it will be senior qualified dentists who will take the sample (biopsy) and advise that they will receive a follow-up appointment in two weeks for the outcome.

- *'We ask all our patients to attend that appointment with someone so that if you miss or forget any information, there's someone with you as a second memory bank!'*

- *'We will ring you to come in sooner if there are any issues.'*

- Highlight the need for further investigations depending on results (CT).

Support after the appointment

- Provide the patient with a leaflet regarding the biopsy and also ensure that they have a phone number to call if they have any questions.

- Ask if they have any questions – very important to check this!

Example 2

You are a DCT in Oral Surgery, and you have been asked to consent Mr Saunders, a 38-year-old male patient who is due to have a mesioangular impacted mandibular wisdom tooth (LR8) surgically removed due to chronic pericoronitis. The patient has not had any dental treatment previously, aside from a small occ-lusal composite filling.

RMH: Patient takes Rivaroxaban once daily in the morning due to previous pulmonary embolism.

SH: Non-smoker, 2 units of alcohol per week and currently works as a self-employed plumber.

DH: Brushes 2x day. Regular attendance at GDP.

OE:

Extra-oral: NAD – Good opening of 45mm and adequate access.

Intra-oral :

Soft tissues show inflamed operculum over the LR8, which is partially erupted and carious. The LR7 is sound. There is no UR8 present.

You note from your OPT radiograph that the LR8 apices are far above the inferior dental nerve, and the risk of injury to this nerve is low.

Question:

The patient attends today for an oral surgery consultation following a referral by his GDP. You are asked to consent for the surgical removal of this LR8 and to book the patient in for treatment.

Answer:

The patient is currently asymptomatic today. However, he wishes to have the tooth removed as it has been very painful. He is worried about the treatment, especially the need for the gum to be cut.

Introduction and rapport building

- Greet the patient and introduce yourself and advise him how you are going to help.

- Check the patient's name, address, and date of birth.

- Ensure the patient understands why he has attended today and inform him that it is just a consultation. *'I understand you have been referred here by your dentist, due to a lower wisdom tooth which has been causing you a lot of trouble.'*

- Collect a short history. *'I have read that this has caused you multiple episodes of pain.'*

- Check medical health and any medications or allergies – although it is stated in the referral letter, you have not personally seen this patient previously and, therefore, you must ask. You could simply ask *'other than the previous pulmonary embolism, do you have any other medical conditions? Are you taking anything other than Rivaroxaban?'*

- Note that with this medication it is important to establish when the patient takes this. *'Am I correct to say you just take this in the morning?'*

- Check smoking and alcohol status (if you suspect other habits, it may be prudent to ask about chewing tobacco, betel nut or paan).

- Check the patient's availability for appointments. *'Are you flexible with the dates you can make the treatment appointment?'*

- Patients who have wisdom teeth removed should be asked about their occupation due to the material impact this may have upon their lifestyle and occupation should the lower lip, chin, or tongue develop anaesthesia from injury to the IDN.

Explain your management

- *'So from looking in your mouth and from taking a full x-ray of the tooth and roots, we can see the tooth has a chronic infection around the gum, causing an inflamed and painful area overlying the tooth. In addition, the area is trapping lots of foods and we can see early decay into the wisdom tooth.'*

- *'Unfortunately, the decay within the tooth is not treatable and is likely to get a lot worse if left, and potentially lead to future problems with the tooth in front.'*

- *'In order to prevent these further problems, we would need to remove the tooth. This would involve numbing the area with local anaesthetic and making a small cut in the gum and possibly loosening some of the bone holding the tooth in place. This way the tooth can be removed in sections, and the gum would then be put back together with dissolvable stitches.'*

The patient informs you that he is worried about the need to cut the gum and have stitches.

Address the patient's concerns

- Anxiety management: Reassure, empathise, and provide the patient with options to manage this.

- *'I can see you are quite worried. This is normal for people who are having teeth removed; however, I can assure you that you will be pain-free throughout the treatment due to the use of strong local anaesthetic.'*

- *'You will not feel any sharpness or pain throughout, but you may feel pressure and hear some buzzing sounds – but this is just the tooth being removed and is normal.'*

- *'The qualified dentist who takes the tooth out will check the area before starting and take their time, so you feel at ease and in control.'*

The patient suggests if there is anything you can do to calm his nerves.

- Explain, without jargon, to the patient the various forms of anxiety control – inhalation, intravenous, and general anaesthetic. *'There are a number of ways we can help control your nerves; these include...'*

- *'Inhalation sedation involves the use of a mask that you wear over your nose. The mask delivers two gases, oxygen and nitrous oxide, which makes you feel relaxed and calms your nerves; you are still awake, and we would still need to provide you with an injection inside the mouth.*

- *'Intravenous sedation involves giving medication through a vein on the back of your hand or arm; this makes you feel sleepy, and you can sometimes forget what has happened. You are still awake but very relaxed and drowsy.'*

- *'General anaesthetic is where you are put completely to sleep, and you are not aware of what is happening. This is also done by giving you medication through a vein.'*

- It is important to outline the advantages, disadvantages, risks, and benefits of each method of anxiety control. These may include:

Inhalation sedation advantages:

1) Least invasive form of sedation (doesn't require to insert needle into vein)

2) No need for escort

3) Rapid onset

4) Offers some analgesia

5) Rapid recovery

Disadvantages:

1) Not good for those who have nasal obstruction

2) Some patients may find it claustrophobic

3) Relies on continual patient reassurance

Intravenous sedation advantages:

1) Provides sedation through the use of medication rather than psychological reassurance (like IHS)

2) Causes anterograde amnesia (forget what has happened after drug is given)

3) Has anticonvulsant properties

Disadvantages:

1) Requires an escort to attend and be with patient for 24 hours post-op

2) Does not produce analgesia

3) Can cause some patients to become more anxious (disinhibition)

4) Need to take day off work following treatment to recover

General anaesthetic advantages:

1) Patient is completely put to sleep

2) Useful for those who are unable to tolerate any treatment awake

3) No memory of the treatment

Disadvantages:

1) Risk of irreversible damage to organs and mortality

2) If no facilities for GA then another referral needed, which may delay time patient receives treatment

3) Must bring an escort

4) May need more time to recover following treatment

5) May require more than one tooth removed – teeth with doubtful prognosis may need to be removed also

   ¤ The patient requests intravenous sedation, so you must ensure that he is able to bring an escort, who is able to accompany the patient throughout treatment and take him home and stay with him for 24 hours. You must ensure that he wears flat shoes, loose clothing, has only a light meal 2 hours before, and avoids alcohol and any recreational drugs.

   ¤ Due to the Rivaroxaban, the patient will need to delay his morning dose (in accordance with SDCEP guidance) and begin this four hours following the bleeding stopping.

The actor agrees to intravenous sedation and wonders if there are any risks when removing the tooth.

Obtain consent

   • There will be a set number of marks available for risks and benefits of the procedure and how you explain these to patients.

- You have already explained the anxiety control; you must explain the benefits and risks of the surgical procedure.

- *'When having any tooth removed, you may experience bleeding, swelling, bruising, post-operative infection and pain (which can be managed with over-the-counter pain-killers). There will also be a need for dissolving stitches, as the gum will be cut. As this is a wisdom tooth, there is a risk of jaw joint pain or dry socket (which is when the blood clot doesn't form or is lost), and you may experience some difficulty opening and closing your mouth afterwards.'*

- It is very important to make patients aware of the risk to the inferior alveolar/dental nerve and lingual nerve when removing any wisdom tooth, regardless of whether the risk is low or not.

- *'Within the lower jaw bone is a special nerve that supplies the teeth, gums, lower lip and chin with sensation. This nerve runs underneath the roots of your wisdom tooth. From your x-ray, we can see that this nerve is not touching the tooth roots but is beneath them, so there is a low risk of bruising to this nerve when the tooth is removed. There is still a risk, but this is low (2 in 100 people). If, however, the nerve is bruised when removing the tooth, this can lead to altered or lost sensation to these areas on the right side only, which may be temporary or permanent.*

- *'On the inner surface of the jaw bone is also an important nerve which supplies the front 1/3 of the tongue with general sensation: touch, pressure, temperature, and taste (chorda tympani). In even fewer patients this may be bruised when the tooth is removed. If this occurs, this can lead to altered or lost sensation and taste to these areas on the right side of the tongue, which may be temporary or permanent.'*

Follow up and aftercare

- Explain that on the day the patient's escort must be present for the treatment to be done under intravenous sedation.

- Reassure the patient that there will be a senior qualified dental surgeon present when removing the tooth, to ensure the procedure runs smoothly.

- Explain that it is useful to have some paracetamol at home to ease the post-operative pain.

- As this is non-urgent, aim to book appointments around the patient and the escort and aim to schedule an appointment date today so they know when they can take time off for the treatment.

- Due to the use of anticoagulants, it may be best to book an appointment early on in the day so that the patient can be monitored and predictable haemostasis can be achieved.

- Print an appointment card so the patient does not forget, and advise them you can call them prior to the day to check they can still make it.

Support after the appointment

- Provide the patient with a leaflet regarding the treatment and sedation and also ensure that they have a phone number to call if they have any questions.

- Advise that on the day of treatment, they will need to wait until they are steady on their feet and approved by a clinician before leaving the hospital.

- They must be informed that for 24 hours following treatment they must not drive, operate machinery, return to work, sign legal documents or even browse online. Make the patient aware that all of these instructions will be provided to their escort on the day, including aftercare for the extraction.

- Ask if they have any questions – very important to check this!

Example 3

You are a DCT in paediatric dentistry and have been asked to see Charlie, a 4-year-old child, and gain consent for extractions of all deciduous carious molars.

RMH: Patient is fit and well, has been taking Calpol.

SH: Lives with mother at home.

DH: Brushes 1x week, poor attender.

Extra-orally – NAD.

Intraoral examination reveals:

STE – NAD

Hard tissue: All eight deciduous molars are carious and unrestorable.

There are no systemic signs or symptoms.

The patient is a healthy weight and height for general anaesthesia.

Question:

The actor here is the patient's mother, here to see you today for a consultation, and you will need to advise her that these teeth need removing. You must confirm the treatment plan and form of anxiety control for the child and obtain consent for this treatment.

Answer:

The actor is very resistant about her child having a GA and will continue to ask questions to prevent this procedure. Your aim is to reassure the parent about her concerns, gain informed consent for GA for the removal of these teeth and then establish a prevention plan for the patient to prevent reoccurrence of dental caries.

Introduction and rapport building

- Greet the patient's mother in an open and friendly manner.

- Introduce yourself and advise her how you are going to help.

- Confirm the relationship to the child – *'Can I just check, are you Charlie's mum?'*

- Recap the history to ensure the mother is aware of the pain – *'I understand from Charlie that he's been in a lot of pain and hasn't been able to sleep. How long have you noticed this for?'*

- Check medical health and any medications or allergies – this is important as you are consenting Charlie for a GA.

- Check social status – who will be coming with Charlie when he has treatment?

Explain your management

- *'So I've had a look at Charlie's teeth, and I can see that he's got a lot of decayed baby teeth which will need to be removed to free him of pain and infection.'*

Address the mother's concerns

- The mother may start to ask you about saving the teeth at this point:

  - Explain to her that the decay has gone through the centre of the tooth into the root and, therefore, they cannot be saved.

  - 'If these teeth are to remain and the infections remain, it can lead to damage to the underlying adult teeth in the long term, which means that when they erupt, they may be damaged or exhibit some irregularities.'

- The mother may become concerned about the GA:

  - Explain that you will be able to remove all teeth effectively whilst Charlie is asleep as he may find it difficult to tolerate this procedure awake.

  - Explain that you want to minimise the trauma to him and would prefer to ensure he is as comfortable as possible.

- Patient anxiety: Aim to seek why it is that the mother is worried.

The actor may ask questions related to the plan.

Typical questions may include:

'Are there any other options?'

- Explain that you won't be able to fill the teeth as they cannot be saved.

- Explain that under 5-year-olds are eligible for GA only and are not old enough yet for sedation.

- Explain that he will not be compliant to have 8 teeth out under LA.

'What is the risk of death?'

- *'There is always a risk of mortality with any GA procedure, and it is roughly 1 in 400,000; however, the anaesthetist will be able to discuss this with you in further detail. Fortunately, Charlie has no complex health conditions, which means he is less likely to have complications during and after surgery.'*

Obtain consent

There will be a set number of marks available for risks and benefits of the procedure and how you explain these.

- *'Today we will be getting your consent for the removal of 8 baby molar teeth from Charlie under general anaesthetic.'*

You should mention to the mother:

- This procedure will last around 30–45 minutes in total.

- The benefits of the procedure are to free him from pain and infection.

- *'The standard risks of the surgical procedure are: pain, bleeding, swelling, bruising, dry socket (infection of the tooth socket) and damage to underlying or adjacent teeth. Because we are taking out teeth earlier than they are due to fall out (exfoliate), the adult teeth may come through at different times and in different positions, which may mean there is a greater chance Charlie may need orthodontic treatment in future.'*

- *'He may wake up with stitches in the area, which will be dissolvable, and you won't have to worry about coming back to have them removed through another procedure. These help reduce the bleeding.'*

- *'Even though we will be doing the procedure under GA, we will still give Charlie some local anaesthetic in his mouth so that when he wakes up, he's not in pain. However, this can increase the chance that he may rub or bite the numbed area without realising. He will need to be supervised until the anaesthetic wears off.'*

- Explain the risks of a GA briefly but reassure them that the anaesthetist will see them prior to the surgery to go through these in more detail:

  - *'There is a small chance your child may have a reaction to the GA. Approximately 1 in 20,000 children may develop a severe allergy to the anaesthetic used.'*

  - *'The anaesthetist will talk to you about different ways of putting Charlie to sleep and what to expect when he wakes up.'*

You realise that the mother may struggle to make the appointment due to the management of other children and taking time off work.

Follow up and aftercare

- Reassure the patient that you can book a date for the procedure that suits them. Take into consideration that Charlie attends school and offer an appointment during the school holidays if possible and check that it suits her other responsibilities.

- Print an appointment card for the pre-operative appointment and schedule the surgery date.

- This is where you discuss the long-term management for Charlie to prevent such a situation arising again.

  ❑ Refer to the Delivering Better Oral Health Dental ToolKit

  ❑ Stress the importance of good oral hygiene, especially because children need to be put into good habits for when their adult teeth come through

  ❑ Offer a leaflet on how to look after baby teeth

  ❑ Discuss the importance of fluoride therapy and regular visits to the dentist in future

Support after the appointment

- Provide the mother with a leaflet about GA with all the information regarding when to stop eating and drinking, etc. Ensure that they have a phone number to call if they have any questions.

- Ask if they have any questions – very important to check this!

<u>Example 4</u>

You are a DCT in general duties, and you have been seeing patients on an oral surgery local anaesthetic MOS list. Your next patient, Tony Williams, has been incorrectly booked onto your list when he should have been booked for intravenous sedation for the simple extraction of an over-erupted UL8 exacerbating the pericoronitis on the LL8.

RMH: Patient is fit and well, non-smoker, no alcohol consumption.

SH: He is a self-employed mortgage advisor.

DH: Good oral hygiene but fears the dentist, particularly the sound of drilling.

OPT shows a conical simple root form of the UL8 away from the maxillary sinus, which you feel is a simple extraction.

Question:

You must speak to the patient, advise him of the error, and manage the situation.

Answer:

The patient has taken time off to attend this visit and has been building up to having this tooth removed. He has also brought his wife, who has also taken time off to attend. The patient is very frustrated that this appointment has been incorrectly scheduled.

Introduction and rapport building

- Greet the patient in an open and friendly manner

- Introduce yourself, advising the patient who you are and what your job role is

- Check the patient's name, address, and date of birth

- Establish why the patient has attended today and confirm their understanding. *'I understand you have been scheduled to have a sedation appointment for the removal of your upper left wisdom tooth.'*

- Collect a short history and obtain whether this tooth is symptomatic. (A symptom-free tooth may be left (and treatment postponed), but it would be prudent to manage a tooth which is causing the patient significant symptoms). *'Is this tooth currently painful today?'*

Today you are informed the patient is not in pain but just wants this tooth removed before it flares up.

- Check medical health and any medications or allergies. You may quickly run through this by asking, *'Am I correct in saying that you have no medications, allergies, or health conditions?'* This is much better than asking, *'Are you fit and well?'* as a patient's perception of this may be different to yours, and this is unspecific.

Explain the mistake and apologise

- You must admit to the error which has been caused, and inform the patient of this. The examiners will be looking to see whether you have demonstrated duty of candour.

- Duty of candour is a regulation set out in the Health and Social Care Act 2008 (Regulated Activities) and entails informing patients, and those that are acting lawfully on behalf of patients, when things go wrong in a truthful manner, and providing an apology and reasonable support.

- It is also important that you do not blame others for this error, as this may create a negative impression of the department or hospital and put the team to disrepute.

- *'I know that you have been awaiting this appointment since last month when you attended for assessment; I am, however, extremely sorry to inform you that you have been incorrectly booked onto today's appointment diary which involves taking teeth out without sedation but with just local anaesthetic alone.'*

Following informing the patient of this news, you find he is very frustrated as both he and his wife have taken time off work to be here.

Manage the frustration

- You should empathise with the patient over his disappointment and advise that you will do everything you can today to help.

- Assure the patient that this error will be highlighted to the clinical bookings team so this does not happen again to them or any other patients.

- Apologise sincerely to the patient and acknowledge his frustration.

- Advise the patient that you will aim to seek a full explanation as to why this has occurred and that you will actively chase this up so that an explanation is reached.

You note that the patient is increasingly irritated that this appointment has been a waste of time.

Offer the patient a resolution

- Explain to the patient that you have various options to help:

- You may attempt to see if there are any free slots or DNAs where other patients may have cancelled or not attended, so that the patient can be seen by a colleague who has an IV sedation list running today.

- You may be able to see if a colleague can see this patient if they have finished treating a patient on an existing IV sedation list.

- (It is worth mentioning to the patient that although you may try, there is no guarantee that a slot may be available today).

- If this is not possible, you may offer to remove the tooth today under LA alone. Here it is important to gauge the patient's anxiety level and explain that the procedure is relatively simple, and you can use topical numbing cream to dampen the feeling of the needle. Some patients may have a false perception of what the treatment may involve; therefore, it is fundamental to clearly explain the procedure and reassure the patient that you will take your time, take frequent breaks, and ensure he is in control.

- The final option would be to offer to rebook the patient for IV sedation.

  ¤ In doing so you should inform the patient that you will ensure that they are booked onto the correct list by personally speaking to the administrator yourself.

Following discussion of the options, the patient wishes to be rebooked so that he can be treated with intravenous sedation when he is more relaxed!

Goodwill gesture

- As a gesture of goodwill, aim to ensure the patient is prioritised and book him in for treatment ASAP. Ensure that the patient's appointment is convenient for him and his escort as they have both had to take a day off to attend today.

- Advise the patient that you will move him to the top of the cancellation list so that if there are any earlier appointments, you can call him.

- Aim to book the appointment today so the patient and his wife know when to take time off work.

Ensure that you take their contact details so that if there are any earlier appointments, you can contact them.

Follow up and aftercare

- Print an appointment card so they do not forget, and advise them you can call them prior to the day to check they can still make it.

- Advise them that it will be a relatively simple extraction, which should not take more than 30 minutes.

- Advise that if there are any further problems with this tooth, in the meantime before the appointment, to visit their normal dentist for emergency pain relief or call NHS 111 if unable to obtain an appointment.

Support after the appointment

- Provide the patient with a leaflet regarding the treatment and also ensure that they have a phone number to call if they have any questions.

- Ask if they have any questions? Very important to check this!

Situational judgement test (SJT)

Ranking

1) You are on a pre-theatre ward round to check all the surgical patients that starts late. The registrar takes a patient through a rushed consent process for the removal of both lower 8's under GA. The only thing that was discussed and written on the paper consent was pain, bleeding, infection, and swelling.

a. Talk over the registrar, informing the patient of the risks that they have left out to ensure a more detailed consent process

b. Wait until the end of the ward round – go back and re-consent the patient more thoroughly

c. Wait until the registrar has gone to see another patient and spend a couple of minutes with the patient to go through a more thorough consent process

d. Leave it as it is – as the risk of paraesthesia is low

e. Ask the fifth-year student who is shadowing to take consent, as they also have noticed that the registrar has missed to consent for paraesthesia and altered taste.

C, B, A, E, D.

C – Here you are ensuring that the patient is fully informed whilst also being considerate and not undermining the registrar.

B – This option ensures that the patient fully consents for treatment; however, you are delaying this process, and there is a risk that the theatre staff will send for the patient, and then it might be hard to catch them in time to consent more thoroughly.

A – This may undermine the registrar; however, it is in the patient's best interest, and the registrar would accept they have made a poor attempt at consenting the patient. This is less preferred to option B, where you are not undermining your colleague and are able to re-consent the patient promptly.

E – This is less ideal as you cannot guarantee that the fifth-year student will ensure that the patient receives all the information, risks, benefits, and alternatives. However, it is better than option D, which would mean the patient is taken to theatre without being aware of all the risks, and therefore, consent would not be valid.

D – This is not in the patient's best interest, is deplorable practice, and is considered negligent.

2) You are a DCT 1 on call and preparing to suture a large eyebrow laceration in a busy OMFS casualty clinic. As you begin, your bleep goes off, and you are informed there are another two casualties waiting. You need help and ask the registrar and consultant. However, they are both busy in theatre. You find that this repeatedly happens, and there just isn't enough senior support.

    a. Continue as you are and hope that nothing goes wrong

    b. Talk to another DCT 1 and ask them for help

    c. Contact a DCT 2, 3 or middle grade and ask them for advice and help

    d. Raise your concern directly with the consultant that you feel there isn't enough support from them

    e. Talk to your Educational Supervisor regarding the lack of senior support

C, B, E, D, A

C – It would be appropriate to ask someone senior first for help; however, if this is not possible because they are busy, the next level up from DCT 1 would be most appropriate. A large eyebrow laceration can wait if you feel you need help and advice.

B – Ideally you should aim to contact someone senior. Speaking to a DCT may be helpful, but given they are the same level of experience as you, they may not be able to offer help.

E – it is important if you feel this is a repeating problem to contact your Education Supervisor initially as they can then raise issues further with a consultant.

D – Consultants are usually very busy with their own clinics and theatre list, therefore, speaking to your education supervisor first is more appropriate.

A – Patient safety is paramount, especially during DCT. Therefore when you feel the treatment is beyond your capability or you feel that harm potentially may result from your actions, it is prudent to ask for help.

3) You are on call; it has been hectic, and you have just had time to have some lunch, and the nurse comes to tell you that a patient who is 5 days post-op for a major head and neck case is scoring a NEWS of 7 and does not look at all well. You are alone on the ward as the only maxillofacial DCT and have not come across this scenario before.

a. Ask your FY2 ENT colleague who shares the ward with you and is also on their break to come with you to assess the patient

b. Go straight to the patient, assess them with ABCDE, start them on O2 and contact the registrar

c. Tell the nurse you will see the patient after you have had a break as you're exhausted

d. Tell the nurse to find someone else as you're having a break

e. Call the registrar immediately

B, A, E, D, C

B – Regardless if you have not seen this before, it is your responsibility to manage your patients. The most appropriate option would be to assess the patient, start them on oxygen to help, and then contact the registrar using the acronym SBAR (Situation, Background, Assessment, Recommendations of management).

A – Overall, the patient is the responsibility of maxillofacial and not ENT; however, recruiting an FY2 junior doctor will help in the assessment of the medically unwell patient. By first managing the patient with the FY2 doctor, you may not need to call upon the registrar.

E – You should not instantly call upon the registrar, as they will be far more able to help if you have more information to tell them other than an unwell patient with a NEWS score of 7. Option A is preferred to this as at least you have someone medically trained with you. The registrar may be busy, and you must manage the situation whilst they make their way to you.

D – This is unprofessional and puts the patient at risk. You may be tired, but this is not an appropriate option, ever. However, it is more appropriate than option C as you are partly addressing the problem and not waiting till after your break.

C – Least preferred option as you are not acting in the patient's interest; inappropriate and unsafe.

4) You are in theatre assisting with a busy minor oral surgery general anaesthetic list. The consultant starts to operate on the left mandibular third molar; however, you are confident that it is the lower right mandibular molar that is to be removed only.

a. Stop the treatment and ask the theatre staff who are not scrubbed to check the consent

b. Inform the consultant you believe that they are operating at the wrong site

c. Drop the sterile instruments on the floor, therefore forcing a break in the surgery

d. Stop the treatment and read the patient's clinical records yourself to ensure that the correct extraction is being performed

e. Ask the consultant to pause and for the team to perform another WHO checklist to ensure safe site surgery.

E, A, B, D, C

E – You are acting promptly to stop the treatment, preventing the consultant causing any harm, and the staff can perform a full WHO checklist to prevent missing out information; this would be most appropriate as this will check the patient details and consent

A – Here you are acting to prevent harm and using initiative to ask another staff member who is not scrubbed to check the consent form

B – This option informs the consultant of the problem but does not ensure that they stop. With option A you are telling the consultant to stop

D – Although you are acting to prevent harm, you also unnecessarily have to remove your gloves to check the notes, whereas you could have asked a colleague to do this (Option A)

C – Dropping the sterile instruments on the floor may not stop the consultant, and they may continue with treatment expecting the nursing staff to replace instruments. Also, this prolongs the treatment time and incurs additional costs as more instruments are needed.

5) A fellow OMFS DCT 1 is always late for clinics and misses the majority of the morning ward round. You find this places more pressure and workload on you. They inform you at lunch that they are not enjoying their post and wish to return to general dental practice once their post finishes.

a. Remind your fellow DCT that they have a duty of care to the patients, and until they finish the post, they must behave professionally and contribute to good teamwork

b. Tell them that if they dislike their post they should inform their educational supervisor about their concerns

c. Discuss with your DCT colleague further why they are not enjoying their post

d. Speak to their educational supervisor of your concerns

e. Speak to your educational supervisor of your concerns

C, A, B, E, D

C – Exploring their concerns may help to understand more about their behaviour. Working and supporting colleagues is important to ensure positive moral and good teamwork.

A – You must remind your colleague that it is important to be part of the team as this is placing a burden on you and other colleagues and is putting patient safety at risk.

B – Advising them that they should speak to their education supervisor is important as they may be able to discuss help and support. It is important not to assume that your colleague is struggling due to work-related issues; there may be other underlying problems.

E – Telling your educational supervisor is essential as their behaviour is placing more strain on your workload. From here, your educational supervisor may escalate this to the appropriate staff members.

D – Ideally you should aim to approach your own supervisor, as this is your first line of contact for any work-related issues. However, if no improvements are made, it then may be appropriate to contact their supervisor.

6) You are two weeks into your DCT 1 post and have been timetabled to perform an incisional biopsy for a suspected fibro-epithelial polyp. You have read about these but do not feel confident to perform this alone. You are the only DCT 1 on clinic, and your other DCT colleagues seem to be busy.

> a. Inform the patient this is a simple procedure, but advise them that you may get help from another colleague throughout the treatment

> b. Attempt to complete the treatment alone as you are aware it is a very busy clinic and your colleagues are busy

> c. Bring the patient in, provide anaesthesia and try to find help from a senior colleague if you are struggling

d. Discuss the case with a senior clinician and advise them that they may need to call upon their help if you are struggling

e. Discuss the case with a senior clinician and kindly ask them to perform the treatment whilst you observe them

E, D, A , C , B

E – You are only two weeks in and have not performed biopsy previously; therefore, in the interest of patient safety and learning, you ought to watch over a senior colleague initially.

D – This is the next safest option as you have discussed the case and are aware when to stop to prevent harm and a senior is informed of when they can help.

A – By informing the patient, you are putting their interest first and reassuring them that calling upon colleagues is normal for their treatment.

C – Option C is worse than option A as although you have given LA, there may not be a senior clinician present and, therefore, you may have given invasive LA to find you have to abandon the procedure if you are unsure how to proceed.

B – This is the least favourable as patient safety is at risk and no other staff members have has been informed should they need to help you out.

7) You are 3 months into your oral surgery DCT 1 post and are scheduled onto the MOS DCT list. You notice that the 9am patient is due to have a horizontally impacted mandibular third molar removed under local anaesthesia, which you feel may be challenging as you have only removed simple mesio-angular impacted third molars previously. It is now 9.15am, and your supervising consultant colleague has not arrived. Your DCT colleagues also appear to be busy with their own patients.

a. Discuss the case with a senior clinician and explain how you would approach this and draw out a surgical plan

b. Advise the patient that there is a delay, and apologise for the wait, informing them you will see them once your colleague appears

c. Proceed with the treatment beginning by providing anaesthesia and then consulting a colleague if you begin to require assistance

d. Ask a nurse to call your consultant and inform them of your situation whilst you provide the patient with anaesthesia

e. Let your DCT 2 colleague see this patient as you feel that they have more surgical experience

B, A, D, C, E

B – Advising the patient of the delay shows initiative and courtesy, and by acknowledging the patient and being honest, you are demonstrating probity.

A – If you are not confident about the treatment, you need to take actions which do no harm. Seeking more information from a senior clinician and drawing a surgical plan will give you far more insight into how to go about treatment. This demonstrates proactive behaviour and also primes the senior clinician to your level of confidence.

D – By asking your nurse to contact the supervising consultant of your situation you are being proactive in managing the situation. Firstly, you are advising the consultant of the need for their help, but you are also exhibiting good time management skills by delegating this to your nurse while you provide anaesthesia, so the patient is not kept waiting.

C – Option D is preferred as with this option if you proceed and become stuck, you may not find a free clinician to get help. In addition, there is a risk of you doing harm if you are unsure of when to stop. If a suitable clinician cannot be found, then the patient will have been given invasive local anaesthesia for the treatment to be abandoned.

E – You are already aware that your colleagues are busy; therefore, it would not be good teamwork to place this onto their list. This would put additional workload on them, increasing the chance of error if they feel time pressured. In addition, the patient would have to wait much longer. As a DCT you are responsible for your own patients and getting help with a patient is better than placing an additional burden onto your colleagues.

8) Every Thursday afternoon you work with a senior colleague on a junior DCT surgical list. You begin to notice that if you are longer than 30 minutes with a surgical tooth removal, they will interrupt and complete your treatment to ensure that they can get home early. You feel this is frustrating, as you are not improving your surgical and suturing skills.

a. Speak to your colleague and explain that you feel rushed and are not benefiting from the learning experience

b. Speak to your other DCT 1 colleagues to see whether they have noticed this behaviour

c. Contact your educational supervisor to explain the situation

d. Reflect upon this in your portfolio with an aim to increase your clinical speed

e. Speak to your line manager to see if you can be booked onto another list to avoid this particular clinician

A, D, C, B, E

A – Speaking to your colleague and honestly discussing your feelings in a constructive and non-confrontational way will aim to help them understand how they are impacting your learning. Taking action is important to allow you to learn, and approaching the colleague is your first step.

D – Reflecting on this learning event is important and a critical part of self-development. Reflections will help you analyse the event, identify why a particular event has occurred, and formulate a plan to improve and prevent this reoccurring.

C – Option D was preferred to this as approaching your educational supervisor straight away is unlikely to resolve the situation immediately. If this is a clinical issue, where it is a procedure-based learning event, your supervisor will most likely encourage you to reflect on this event first. If after reflecting and speaking to the individual you feel you still are struggling, then it would be prudent to seek advice from your supervisor.

B – Gathering information from your fellow DCTs is useful; however, this would not do anything to address the issue immediately. Speaking to DCTs about your clinical issue is not likely to improve things.

E – Going to your line manager is the worst option. This is a very drastic decision and asking to be moved to another clinician would involve rearranging all the timetables and also affecting another individual who you switch with. Here there is no self-reflection, and a logical approach has not been followed.

9) A patient has been booked to see you in the oral medicine clinic for investigation of a suspected lump on the palate. From reading the notes, you are aware this may simply be a palatal torus. You are aware that the patient's appointment has been cancelled and rescheduled twice, and they are very frustrated. When you call the patient in, they are verbally abusive to you.

a. Explain to the patient that it was the receptionists' fault, and they are responsible for the delay

b. Advise the patient if they continue to be abusive you will call security

c. Refuse to see the patient as you feel threatened

d. Explain to the patient you are sorry to hear that their appointments have been rescheduled and you will aim to determine why this has occurred

e. Call security as you are convinced that this patient will not calm down

D ,B ,E ,C ,A

D – Empathising with your patient is an important aspect of communication and customer service, and an appropriate thing to do when a patient is frustrated. Also, by explaining that you will seek further information about why this has occurred, you are acknowledging the patient's frustration with the service.

B – It is not acceptable to be abused by any patients, and therefore, the patient should be firmly but kindly reminded of the rules of the hospital. If you feel threatened, you have a right to stop treatment.

E – If despite your efforts to calm the patient down you feel the patient may continue, calling security may be necessary to prevent putting you, your colleague, and other patients in danger.

C – Immediately refusing to see the patient is not wise, as this may aggravate the situation further and lead to harm to you or a complaint. It is important to try to calm the patient down initially; however, if the patient continues to be abusive, you have a right to refuse to see the patient.

A – Blaming other staff members is not professional and can lead to negative impacts on others unnecessarily. This is dishonest and will not improve the situation. This is unprofessional and not a sign of good teamwork.

10) You arrive at your Monday morning LA oral surgery clinic and notice that the first patient has been incorrectly booked in. Reading their records, you observe that they were due for surgical removal of their mandibular third molar under intravenous sedation but have been booked onto your local anaesthetic surgical list.

a. Apologise to the patient and reschedule their appointment for the next available intravenous sedation session

b. Apologise to the patient, informing them of the mix-up, and offer the patient the option of removal today under local anaesthetic alone

c. Inform the patient of the error and speak with your senior colleague to see whether there are any available slots today for intravenous sedation

d. Don't inform the patient of the error but proceed to take the tooth out under intravenous sedation using your colleagues' bay

e. Explain to the patient that if they wish to have the tooth out under intravenous sedation, they may attend a private dental clinic

C, B, A, E, D

C – Informing the patient of the error demonstrates probity and duty of candour. In addition, speaking to your colleague to see whether there are any free slots available shows initiative and can potentially save the patient from returning. There can sometimes be DNAs, and so this shows very proactive behaviour.

B – Apologising to the patient and providing them with an alternative is the next best option as although they have been booked in incorrectly, you are still managing the situation by offering a solution.

A – Here you are showing probity by apologising and offering to rebook at the next available date. However, option B is preferred as the patient is offered an alternative on the day, preventing them from returning and saving them time. With this option, they still need to rebook and spend time travelling to the appointment.

E – It is not helpful to explain to the patient that if they wish to have intravenous sedation today, they can do this privately. The patient has already been treatment planned for removal at the hospital. Therefore, this would not be a suitable suggestion.

D – Here you are using your colleagues' bay for treatment, thereby delaying their own patients who have been booked for sedation. In addition, you are potentially delaying your own list, as sedation will take longer than local anaesthesia alone.

Best three answers

1) A type II diabetic patient attends A&E with a buccal space abscess, moderate trismus, and pyrexia – their first language is Punjabi. The family member who attends with the patient says they can translate – you plan to admit this patient on IV antibiotics with the likelihood that the patient will need to go to theatre for I&D and removal of the source of infection. The hospital translator cannot attend for at least 3 more hours, as they are very busy.

a. Use the family member to translate the plan

b. Whilst the family member is there, ask them to translate whilst you consent the patient

c. Ask your DCT colleague who speaks Punjabi to communicate with the patient

d. Wait 3 hours until the translator is free, then talk to the patient

e. Use Google translate on your smartphone to consent the patient

f. Use the family member to translate and then consent to save time

g. Explain as best as you can using images and get the patient to sign the consent

h. Continue your other jobs until the translator arrives

A, C, D

A – This is appropriate to explain the plan; however, for consent it is prudent you use a hospital translator to ensure all information is being communicated accurately.

B – Inappropriate for the family member to be used for consent.

C – Another good option, however, only if your colleague is fluent in Punjabi.

D – At present this is not an immediate emergency; we can wait for the hospital translator to consent the patient .

E – Unreliable source for translation.

F – Inappropriate as the family member may not translate exactly what you want the patient to know.

G – You will not be aware of whether the patient has understood the information.

H – This is least appropriate as you may forget or the other jobs may go beyond 3 hours

2) You are a maxillofacial DCT at a busy District General Hospital, and you keep noticing that patients with suspected mandibular fractures are only getting an OPG performed. You have explained to the radiology team that two radiographic views must be obtained for diagnosis of fracture in plain film. Despite you asking multiple times for a PA mandible as well as an OPG, the radiology team continues to only provide an OPG.

   a. Approach your consultant and advise him of the situation, asking him to talk to the radiology team

   b. Perform an audit of the radiographic views being produced and present this to the departmental meeting to implement changes

   c. Ask the radiology team directly to give an explanation as to why they do this

   d. Accept that this will not change and assess mandibular fractures with the use of an OPG only

   e. Attempt to request an OPG with an OM view to determine whether they are able to produce this view

   f. Contact your colleagues to ask whether they are experiencing this problem also

   g. Explain to the radiology department that you will make a complaint to the management team if this does not improve

    h.   Take the radiographs yourself as you will know that the correct views have been produced

A, B, C

A – A senior would likely have more of an impact on the radiology team.

B – Gold standard and could be used to help the department provide the acceptable level of care.

C – This will allow you to understand their reasoning, and you can then deal with the problem more efficiently.

D – Inappropriate as it is highly likely fractures will be missed with only one 2D image.

E – Inappropriate exposure for the given clinical scenario.

F – Although this may be useful in gathering further anecdotal evidence, it will not address the issue directly.

G – This is antagonistic and can lead to a breakdown in relationship.

H – As a busy DCT 1, you will be busy with other, potentially more serious jobs, therefore, by taking the radiograph you will be compromising other ill patients.

3) You are on a biopsy clinic, and the consultant has said to biopsy an ulcer on the labial mucosa of a 25-year-old teacher. It has the appearance of minor RAS, you are confident of the diagnosis from the appearance and history and believe this is not the appropriate first special investigation that is required. What do you do?

    a.   Take full blood count, haematinics and liver and renal function tests as you feel this is the best management

b.   Discuss with your consultant why they want this to be done

c.   Explain to the consultant you think this would not be appropriate first line management

d.   Do nothing as you do not feel sure about the treatment, and rebook the patient for a day when there is a different consultant

e.   Talk to a different senior and explain you think this might not be appropriate

f.   Explain to the patient you feel that the consultant may have got patients confused and prescribe Difflam mouthwash

g.   Seek advice from a DCT 2 colleague you work with

h.   As you are unsure, let the patient be seen by a staff grade

B, C, E

A – You should aim to seek advice prior to conducting an investigation when unsure, as these tests may have already been done initially.

B – There may be something more that you do not know, which may explain why the consultant wants to do it; they will be happy for you to express your intuition.

C – Approaching the consultant, in a non-confrontational manner, to seek advice demonstrates initiative and being a safe clinician.

D – Although you have done no harm, you have not acted to address this situation, and therefore the patient may be frustrated due to the time and mental preparation they have undergone before the appointment. Also, booking this under another consultant is bad practice as you should not change treatment plan without the consultant's approval.

E – Although it is best to approach your consultant, the next best option is to ask someone else for their opinion. You will show that you are putting the best interests of the patient first, which is good practice. Following this, you will gain confirmation as to whether to proceed or approach your consultant if the senior feels this may not be appropriate.

F – You should not speak ill of your colleagues, especially if you do not know why the patient has been booked in as this could lead to inaccurate accusations.

G – The best person to ask is the consultant as they have asked you to perform this treatment, and the DCT 2 may not know what to do and cannot override the decision of a consultant.

H – The staff grade will likely have a busy list of patients, and the consultant has asked you to perform this. It would be inconsiderate and not 'good teamwork' to leave them with things you are uncertain of.

4) You enter the treatment room of a maxillofacial clinic and see that your DCT colleague is midway through suturing a forehead laceration and nearly finished. You notice in the notes this occurred by falling off a push bike onto gravel. You can see from the armamentarium present that they have not debrided the wound and are only suturing it closed. You know there is a risk of gravel tattoo, as it has not been cleaned properly.

    a. Get the patient's number, and call them later when they have gone that they will need to come back to reopen the wound, debride it, and re-suture

b. Trust that the DCT 1 has already explored visually, and there must have been no gravel within the wound

c. Whilst the patient is present, ask your colleague whether they have cleaned the wound and thrown away the cleaning armamentarium

d. Ask your colleague to stop, take them into a separate room and ask whether they have cleaned the wound and thrown away the cleaning armamentarium

e. Tell your education supervisor of your concern before the patient leaves

f. Inform your DCT colleague after, that their patient may have gravel tattoo

g. Discuss your colleague's mistake to the consultant as this should have been managed better

h. Discuss this with your colleague's education supervisor once you have finished your duties

C, D, E

A – There is no guarantee you can contact the patient, this is not appropriate, and you should deal with it immediately.

B – Inappropriate and not addressing your concerns.

C – It would be better to try and ask the colleague whilst the patient is not present. However, it deals with the situation and makes the patient aware there may be a problem. It is not ideal but is in the best interest of the patient.

D – Ideally best, this way you can manage the situation without undermining anyone and overall the patient benefits.

E – Does not address the situation immediately, but is an option if you feel uncomfortable informing your colleague of their error as you are at the same level as them. Doing this before the patient leaves allows actions to be taken prior to the patient leaving.

F – Inappropriate as this may not be true, and you have actioned this after the patient has left.

G – You should not make judgements about your colleague without evidence, and the consultant is not the first person you should contact if you have concerns.

H – Not appropriate as you first do not know for certain whether the gravel was removed; therefore, you should aim to speak to your colleague first to understand the situation.

5) You are busy on the ward; it has been 3 hours, and your DCT colleague who is timetabled for the ward is missing. He returns and says he was in theatre because there was an interesting case. In the meantime, you have been very busy on your own and could have really used the extra hands to do the ward jobs. Because of this, there are about 3 hours' worth of jobs left and it's 3pm.

    a. Explain that despite more interesting things going on in the hospital, your colleague has their own duties. Share the remaining jobs that they were meant to do, so that the workload is halved

    b. Tell your colleague that they owe you 3 hours of work. Tell them that they must stay whilst you go home

    c. Join your colleague in theatre as you agree it is more interesting and will get more surgical experience

    d. Discuss with your educational supervisor how you feel about your colleague's behaviour

e.   Discuss with your colleague that this is not acceptable and explain they may find time outside their clinical hours to observe treatment

f.   Discuss this with your colleague's supervisor

g.   Speak to the consultant who was in theatre to ensure this does not happen again

h.   Encourage your colleague to speak to the OMFS consultant if they are interested in that area of surgery

A, D, E

A – This is what should have happened before your colleague's disappearance.

B – You have a duty to care for patients on the ward; it is therefore not appropriate for you to leave, and this is the same as your colleague going to theatre when not timetabled for it.

C – You have responsibility for patients on the ward. Therefore, this is least appropriate.

D – Speaking with your educational supervisor is another appropriate option as they can escalate this to their supervisor if required.

E – By speaking with your colleague and addressing the problem directly, you may be able to prevent this occurring again.

F – You should aim to speak to your own supervisor initially as they can escalate this to the correct individuals.

G – The consultant should only be approached if, after speaking to your colleague and your education supervisor, this behaviour persists.

H – This is not the most appropriate choice as all DCTs have dedicated responsibility and cannot observe surgery whilst on ward duty.

6) A patient you have just finished treating under intravenous sedation is becoming increasingly anxious and irritable in recovery, as they just want to go home. Your nurse informs you of the situation as she feels they are getting aggressive.

- a. Inform the patient that they are disturbing other patients and making them feel uncomfortable

- b. Empathise with the patient and explain that you can see they are anxious

- c. Explain to the patient the more they worry, the longer recovery will take

- d. Advise the nurse to listen to the patient's concerns and report back to you

- e. Explain gently to the patient the importance of recovering before leaving the clinic

- f. Explain to the patient that they cannot leave

- g. Further sedate the patient so that they are less anxious

- h. Advise the patient's escort to reassure the patient and calm them down

B, D, E

A – This can further irritate patients and make them feel frustrated as they are not being listened to.

B – By empathising with the patient, you will aim to reduce their anxiety and calm them down.

C – This is not productive and may irritate the patient further as you are not helping to resolve their anxiety.

D – Listening skills are essential, especially with patients who show anxiety. From listening to what the patient has to say, you can better manage the situation.

E – You should not let the patient leave until they are stable on their feet; therefore, it is important to convey this to the patient in a non-confrontational manner.

F – Simply explaining that they cannot leave is likely to frustrate the patient more, and therefore option E is more appropriate.

G – Further sedating the patient will make the patient's recovery time longer and would not be advised.

H – It is not the responsibility of the escort to manage the anxious patient.

7) You receive a search warrant request from the police informing you that a patient of yours has been involved in a road traffic accident. They request further access to the patient's dental records to help identify the victim.

a. Inform the police that they will need a court order

b. Ignore their request as you are not certain it is a valid request

c. Write back to the police service asking them to write to the Chief Executive of your healthcare trust

d. Seek consent from the trust Caldicott guardian to disclose confidential information

e. Write back to the police services asking them for further information

f. Speak to your indemnity provider for support

g. Co-operate with the police as regardless of whether they have a court order they have a right to the information

h. Make documented clinical notes of the enquiry and hand over the minimum amount of information needed

F, G, H

A – This is incorrect, and you will be going against the law (see below).

B – This is inappropriate, and you will be going against the law (see below).

C – The police do not require consent from the Chief Executive in this particular situation, as mentioned below.

D – The law states that dental records may be disclosed without patient consent in certain situations where information can be of use to protect the public or prevent a significant risk of harm to patients.

E – This is not true, as mentioned below.

F – Speaking to your indemnity provider is a sensible and appropriate option as they will give you sound unbiased legal advice to protect you and the patient.

G – Under S172 of the Road Traffic Act 1988 you must disclose this information regardless of a court order or search warrant.

H – It is important to document clear, contemporaneous, deta-iled, complete records of what has been asked for.

Ordinarily, the police do not have the right to confidential patient dental records. However, under certain provisions such as Section 172 of the Road Traffic Act 1988, you are required to provide the police with dental records due to the information being of use to protect the public or prevent significant risk of harm to patients.

8) You are an OMFS DCT working on call at a busy casualty clinic. As you enter the waiting room, you notice a 50-year-old male patient being verbally abusive to the reception team. You note that the patients are startled, and as you approach him he is intimidating and demanding.

a. Prescribe analgesics for the patient and send him home

b. Escort the patient to a side surgery and explore how you can help him

c. Ask reception to call the police

d. Assure the patients in the waiting room that they are safe

e. Call security in case the patient becomes more aggressive

f. Speak to the reception team to see if anyone knows this patient

g. Advise the patient that his behaviour is not tolerated, explaining that you cannot treat aggressive patients

h. Speak to the reception team to find out who caused this

B, E, G

A – This is not clinically appropriate as you have not made a diagnosis to prescribe this medication, and this may put the patient's safety at risk if there are any medical contraindications.

B – A sensible option and one where you can explore the patient's concerns to hopefully reduce the patient's frustration.

C – Calling the police prematurely may be unnecessary; if, however, the patient becomes abusive and threatens the safety of other patients, colleagues, and your own, then it may be prudent.

D – As a DCT you should aim to ensure the safety of any victims but also the bystanders. Therefore, you should ensure the safety of other patients by checking on those in the vicinity.

E – Calling security is an appropriate option if you feel the patient's behaviour does not improve and you feel threatened; you should aim to calm the patient down first and then re-assess the situation.

F – This would not help to resolve the situation.

G – You must inform the patient that in this situation, aggression will not help, and it is against hospital policy to treat a patient in this state.

H – You should first ensure the safety of the dental team, and other patients who may be victims of the aggressive patient.

9) A DCT 1 colleague, John, informs you that Sarah, another OMFS DCT 1, has been sleeping throughout her shift in the doctors' mess. You have worked with Sarah previously and are not aware of such behaviour.

    a. Tell John that Sarah must have been on nights and to let her rest

b. Advise that John speaks to Sarah about his concerns, when she awakens

c. Inform your educational supervisor about Sarah's behaviour

d. Advise John to speak to his educational supervisor about this

e. Inform John that this is not your problem and advise him to contact the clinical lead

f. Ask other members of the team whether they have witnessed this behaviour in Sarah

g. Advise John that Sarah should be allowed to sleep as the ward is quiet currently

h. Ask John for any evidence that patient safety is being compromised

B, F, H

A –This comment is not truthful as you are presuming Sarah has been on nights.

B – By speaking to Sarah, John can establish why she has overslept through the shift; it is important not to rush to conclusions or draw false assumptions.

C – Although you should be looking out for your colleagues, option D is more appropriate as John has witnessed this.

D – It is prudent to understand the circumstance before jumping to conclusions. Therefore, John should aim to find out more about the situation and especially if this is a recurrent issue before contacting an appropriate senior for advice.

E – Contacting the clinical leads would be inappropriate as we do not know the truth of the situation; the first port of call is the educational supervisor.

F – Involving others in a colleague's matter can help to gain evidence for you to potentially escalate this further, with an educational supervisor. However, it should be done sensitively to prevent negative team morale.

G – Sarah is on duty and should not be sleeping. If she is ill, she should inform her educational supervisor, and a cover arrangement should be made.

H – A preferred choice as if patient safety is compromised then action can be taken to prevent harm.

Chapter 4

The Dental Portfolio

The dental portfolio will be of particular concern to those app-lying for Dental Core Training 2 and 3 posts. This chapter is dedicated to providing you with essential information to help best prepare you for this station.

The focus of this chapter will be largely on the creation, content and presentation of your dental portfolio itself and not the station. Unlike the 2018 recruitment round, candidates will be asked questions and given chances to provide detail on their dental portfolio. As such, for full details on this new format please refer to the COPDEND website.

What you can expect from this chapter:

1) What exactly the dental portfolio is and why it is an essential tool to impress at interview

2) A step-by-step guide to making your dental portfolio, including the list of items you need!

3) The key structure to enhance your portfolio and add value to your application

4) Tips from experienced interviewers on boosting the presentation of your portfolio

5) Example template documents for each section of your portfolio, allowing you to construct your own portfolio at an accelerated pace!

6) A complete dental portfolio checklist to help you prepare and review your portfolio objectively

What is a dental portfolio?

A dental portfolio is a profile of yourself that exhibits you as an individual to the employer or interviewer. It is a meaningful collection of work that encompasses your experience, achievements, efforts and progress throughout your career to date.

Your portfolio should be tailored to the criteria of the job you are applying to. Interestingly, a clinical experience portfolio is unassumingly collated during DFT through undertaking work-based assessment, ADEPTs and collating a logbook of procedures, often onto an online portal. A true portfolio would not only include these aspects, but also your achievements, qualifications, quality improvement projects, publications, presentation and much more!

Ultimately this is a summary of your entire dental career, often presented in a neatly bound A4 folder, with dividers to separate each aspect of your career to date.

Should I have a dental portfolio?

For Dental Core Training 2 and 3 interviews, it is essential that you have a portfolio to bring with you to the interview.

In the opinion of previous Dental Core Trainees, the portfolio is looked upon as a highly valuable asset. Not only does it evidence previous experiences, cases and additional activities, it provides tangible proof that you are serious about your commitment to dentistry. Therefore, it is highly recommended that you start to build your portfolio as soon as you commence Dental Core Training.

Many foundation dentists and current DCTs may have been using an electronic portfolio rather than a paper-based portfolio. An electronic portfolio is an extremely useful way of collating clinical experiences, reflective logs and recording cases. For current DCTs, the online portfolio (TURAS) provides an array of domains for recording experience and objectively recording progress. Domains such as DOPs, MSFs and CBDs can be input as content for your portfolio.

What is included in a dental portfolio?

The content of a portfolio will largely vary depending upon your experiences and the job you are applying for. A portfolio for a Dental Core Trainee 1 will differ to that of a Dental Core Trainee 3. In addition, the portfolio will vary depending on the type of post applied for; this is because the job criteria are different.

Despite different criteria, a portfolio of evidence will follow a generic format, with certain domains having a greater influence subject upon the job in question. This chapter will focus on clarifying exactly what to include in your portfolio and how to format this, and will also include an example template portfolio and a portfolio checklist. It is worth mentioning that the checklist provided follows a generic format. **In order to secure maximum marks, it is essential to follow the exact instructions detailed by COPDEND for dental portfolio guidance.**

How do I create a dental portfolio?

A well-presented portfolio is not difficult to create; however, it can be time-consuming. It can be easy to print off certificates, pictures of cases or audit results and throw a folder together – but this is not what you should do.

In the views of previous portfolio assessors, a well-organised, easy to navigate and relevant portfolio can make the difference between a highly impactful and engaging portfolio with maximum points, and one that is average.

Items required

1) A4 ring binder, ideally 50mm depth

2) Set of A4 dividers and index such as the 'Leitz style printable index' http://www.leitz.com/en-gb/products/filing ---archiving/ indices---dividers/

3) A4 transparent poly pockets for storage of A4 printouts

4) Colour printer

5) Scissors

The dental portfolio is traditionally presented in a neatly bound A4 folder. The folder is divided into various sub-headings to allow the reader to swiftly flick through the individual sections. The keys to an outstanding portfolio are simplicity, clarity and organisation. According to current practice owners, the most valuable portfolios allow the reader to find what they want quickly and are presented to a high level of quality.

Structuring your portfolio

In order to create a streamlined and logically presented document, the following sub-headings can be utilised:

Front cover: Full name and post-nominal letters with GDC number and what post you are applying for, e.g. DCT 3 applicant.

Inside first page: This will be an index page with labelled dividers clearly corresponding to the sub-headings below. Including dividers allows the reader to quickly flick to each section of your portfolio.

Section 1: Curriculum Vitae – an up-to-date curriculum vitae is essential in forming the first chapter of your portfolio. This should be clear and concise for the interviewer to look through; this will be the same CV that you have sent prior to the interview. As such, a useful technique for presenting your CV, within your portfolio, is to have an initial summary page. This can be a single A4 page that is presented before your CV, allowing the reader to identify the key points from your CV. A template CV Summary has been included here:
https://goo.gl/GEjVFB

Section 2: Undergraduate and Postgraduate Qualifications – This will include your original degree certificate, class of degree and any qualifications achieved such as BSc, MFDS or MJDF. Again, an initial summary page highlighting your key postgraduate and undergraduate qualifications can easily guide the reader. Note, you may not have all of these documents by the time of the interview. See the qualifications template at
https://goo.gl/bvCUn6

Section 3: Prizes and Awards – This section will include any notable achievements you have obtained throughout your undergraduate and postgraduate career pathway. It is prudent to include the title of the award, the awarding body, the reason for the award and the original certificate here. This can really help you stand out amongst your peers!

Remember, the portfolio must be factual and you should avoid fabricating fictitious information. The interviewer may wish to discuss more about these achievements, so it is essential that this information is truthful.

See the prizes and awards template at
https://goo.gl/HouwMc

Section 4: Postgraduate Training, Key Competencies and Experience

Postgraduate training summary

Through Dental Foundation Training you will be expected to carry out numerous supervised cases known as DOPs/DEPs, Mini-CEXs and SLEs. These are all assessments of your level of competence to carry out procedures. These competencies provide evidence for the clinical procedures you state you have carried out. If appropriate and relevant, you can also insert radiographs or photographs (but ensure you have consent first) of the work you have carried out. For example, if you carried out a complex root canal treatment using a specific endodontic rotary system, you can showcase pre-operative and post-operative radiographs of your obturated root canal.

In this section, you should also include your original certificate of completion of Dental Foundation Training or Dental Core Training if you have completed these. This will naturally add credibility to this section and validate your training experience.

Logbook of activity

Throughout your postgraduate training there will be a large amount of information collected regarding your clinical experience. In order to portray this you should aim to include key summary tables from your e-portfolio to make this information more visually attractive.

For clinicians who wish to formulate a logbook of experience, but are beyond DFT, the use of a well-formulated spreadsheet can be used to log clinical cases and reflections. Alternative, the Royal College of Surgeons of Edinburgh have a free online logbook which allows you to record cases in a secure database; see the link at
https://www.elogbook.org/.

Specific dental interests and key competencies

For those DCT 2 or 3s, you will want to list and explain your enhanced or advanced skills in this section. Ideally you should aim to validate your claims; for example, if you have undertaken more complex treatments, then including pre- and post-operative photos will add significance to your skill list. Including high-quality photography, with noticeable improvements in outcomes, is likely to attract the reader as this exhibits the effort you have made to present your acquired skills.

Reflections

Insert meaningful reflections. Do not be shy of inserting reflections on times when you have not performed as well as you would have liked (and also where you have performed well). Reflections are an integral component of your development as a junior member of staff. Transparency and willingness to learn is a key trait of an honest and safe clinician; this allows the assessor to understand your self-awareness and how you are prepared to learn from each case that does not go as planned.

NHS, Google reviews or NHS Family and Friends Tests

Many excellent opportunities arise during DFT, DCT and even during practice to make a great impression with patients. If you have been fortunate enough to receive positive reviews, include screenshot examples, written testimonials or thank-you cards (omitting patient-identifying information) within this section. Portraying these within your portfolio really sells, and offers genuine value in the eyes of the reader.

Ultimately, evidencing positive feedback through these reviews certainly provide tangible proof that patients like you!

NHS services will promote the use of the Family and Friends Test; as such, if you are a current DCT you should aim to collect positive reviews for your portfolio.

Feedback from colleagues

As with patient reviews, the feedback from your colleagues and team members is equally important. Where possible, it is prudent to gather multi-source feedback using a wider range of staff within your current workplace setting. This should include administrative staff, other clinicians, nurses and lab technicians to provide a '360-degree' summary of your abilities to work with the dental team.

See the template for postgraduate training, competencies and experience at
https://goo.gl/nNajJ3

Section 5: Continued Professional Development – This section is important for assessors to see that you have kept up to date with the new eCPD requirements from the GDC. Depending on your experience, you may have built up significant numbers of hours of CPD; therefore this section is likely to be the one with the largest content.

In order to help the reader, it is strongly advised that CPD is presented in a tabular format. This way the information can be browsed efficiently and the reader can find the key information without needing to trawl through masses of text.

As part of the new eCPD, it is important that all CPD is recorded and a reflective log is kept. This aspect of your portfolio will showcase your CPD and should include a reflection of what was learnt, what information was reinforced, how the activity will influence your practice and how this will impact on patient care and quality.

Including original certificates will validate your portfolio and is a necessary requirement for the GDC. Your certificates of attendance can be included in reverse chronological order, after the summary table of CPD activity.

Conferences are a good way to keep up to date with key developments in a field of your interest and they also exhibit your commitment to the profession or specialty.

See the template for CPD at
https://goo.gl/R3pbmH

Section 6: PDP and Career Plan

Since the introduction of the enhanced CPD in January 2018, all dentists must have a Personal Development Plan (PDP). This is a requirement for the GDC, and may be requested by the GDC, should they undertake random sampling of a registrant's records. The PDP provides information on the CPD you plan to undertake during your cycle, the anticipated GDC developmental outcomes achieved from this activity and the expected timeframe you plan to achieve this by.

A PDP can be included within your dental portfolio, so this ensures you are compliant with the GDC but also helps illustrate to the employer your intended learning and developmental plans and how these align with your future career ambitions.

A career plan can really illustrate to the employer your commitment to the profession. Depending on your goals and ambitions, this may vary between a short 5-year plan to a lengthier 10-year plan. It is recommended that you should have a 5-year plan with realistic expectations, including how you aim to reach your milestones.

See an example PDP and career plan here:
https://goo.gl/Anmgpr

Section 7: Quality Improvement Project and Presentations – Quality improvement tools, such as audits, allow you to evaluate the current level of service and make improvements to enhance quality of care. Improvements in health care quality are not exclusive to hospital settings; it is therefore important to demonstrate your experience of quality improvement projects and how they have led to improved outcomes. In addition, if you have any additional presentations, whether they are of a quality improvement project or posters at a local, regional, national or international level, then including these can also add value. If you have done any service evaluations then this will be a place to insert their documentation and their outcomes.

As with all information within your portfolio, you should aim to ensure this information is clear and easy to locate. For example, including a summary table of all the quality improvement projects or key presentations you have undertaken can help the reader ascertain the relevant information with ease. Including copies of the audit presentation, posters and original copies of the programme itinerary (where you have presented) provides strong evidence.

See the clinical governance template at
https://goo.gl/scfTA1

Section 8: Publications (and Research) – Prospective Dental Core Trainees are not expected to have publications or research, as many of the other applicants may not have these either. However, if you do, it is likely to be seen as an added bonus, especially if it is relevant and clear. The reader is unlikely to have time to read through the entire publication or research conducted, so including a summary at the beginning of this section can be useful to highlight the key facts.

See the publications template at
https://goo.gl/1i4k6K

Section 9: Personal Interests – This section of the portfolio can be used to portray your interests and personality outside of work. For example, you may include photographs of you rock climbing, cycling or carrying out charity work, which may or may not be related to dentistry.

See the personal interests template at
https://goo.gl/G6W5LW

What should I exclude from my dental portfolio?

The dental portfolio should aim to include key relevant information that you have undertaken throughout your career to date, that can add value to your application for a DCT role. As such, it is important that quality, rather than quantity, of information is focused on.

Things to avoid:

- Work experience from secondary school – this does not add additional value as you have already completed your dentistry degree and already work as a dentist

- Achievements from primary and secondary school age, e.g. Duke of Edinburgh award, as they will most likely be irrelevant and outdated. However, if they are outstanding achievements, such as competing at national level in a sporting category, they would be appropriate in the "Other" section.

- Only include relevant items that add value to the portfolio. Do not try to increase the size of your portfolio by adding irrelevant pieces of work such as multiple views of a clinical case.

- **Patient identifiable information – It is essential that all images used within your portfolio have received**

appropriate consent for use. In addition, you should exclude any patient identifiable information from reflections, radiographs and case descriptions.

- Fictitious clinical cases, false claims, over-exaggerating your clinical skills – as with all parts of your application, you should demonstrate a high degree of professional probity and avoid any form of false information.

Tips to enhance presentation

A well-presented portfolio reflects on you as an individual. It reflects your presentation skills, effort and enthusiasm for the role.

- **Size**: Consider the size of your ring binder, ensuring it is easy to handle, of high quality and not too large. Remember you will need to carry this in to the interview with you, so it must be practical. If possible, choose a ring binder with a transparent front pocket, which will allow you to include an A4 sheet with your name and GDC number as a front cover.

- **Index for ease**: Ideally, the index should match the headings from your CV, for ease of navigation for the interviewer. However, this is not the only way to present your portfolio, and including additional sub-headings within the portfolio maybe needed to mention aspects that were not feasible to include in your CV – for example, including a career plan and PDP.

- **Poly pockets**: Use punched 'poly pocket' plastic sleeves, two pages back-to-back per sleeve, to prevent the interviewer having to remove and replace multiple pages during the interview.

- **Quality of presentation**: If showcasing previous work through photographs, use photo paper and ensure colour photographs are of a high quality and, needless to state, ensure work you showcase is of the best quality.

- **Have order**: Within each individual section, ensure that the information is presented in reverse chronological order, with the most recent information first, i.e. include most recent CPD first.

- **Clear summary:** For sections where there is significant information, including an initial summary page can help the reader digest the information without needing to read through each page.

- **Consistency:** As with the CV, it is essential to maintain a consistent use of headings, font size and styles. Ensure that this font is the same as the CV and cover letter for completeness.

- **Be personable**: Many principles want to see that you have a personality and will build rapport with patients as a general dental practitioner. One way to demonstrate this is through an "Other" section in your portfolio (see above).

Dental portfolio checklist

The checklist below can be used when compiling your portfolio or when reviewing it. You may wish to provide this checklist to a senior colleague to help with providing objective feedback for your portfolio.

Section 1: Curriculum Vitae	Includes clear summary of dentistry ambitions and reason for application Includes relevant qualifications, employment history and skills Follows a reverse chronological approach Clear and concise information Tailored to the job specification/role	
Section 2: Undergraduate and Postgraduate Qualifications	Includes clear logical order of qualifications, including current status and evidence Mentions name of qualification, awarding body and year awarded	
Section 3: Prizes and Awards	Includes dental and non-dental notable achievements, reason for award, date of award and number of each prizes awarded per year.	
Section 4: Postgraduate Training, Key Competencies and Experience	Name of postgraduate training programme (if applicable) e.g. DFT/DCT/StR Summary of relevant portfolio (if used during period of training e.g. DFT e-portfolio) Includes notable achievements throughout training period and postgraduate employment Includes structured learning events which evidence progression and development Includes colleague and patient feedback Details interests within dentistry, competencies and treatment experience with evidence of cases	
Section 5: Continued Professional Development	Clearly lists the courses attended that are relevant to field of practice; includes reflective note and date of attendance with evidence	

Section 6: PDP and Career Plan	Includes a clearly defined Personal Development Plan with: Explanation of learning, maintenance or developmental need How this learning, maintenance or developmental need relates to your field of practice GDC developmental outcomes this will fulfil How you intend to achieve this unmet need When this will be completed Whether this has been completed Whether a reflection was undertaken following the event Includes a logical and realistic career plan with milestones	
Section 7: Quality Improvement Project and Presentations	Clear summary of quality improvement project with evidence of how changes in practice have been made	
Section 8: Publications (and Research)	Includes any publications including corresponding title, authors, date published and name of publication with evidence	
Section 9: Personal interests	Includes summary of personal interests	
Overall: Presentation quality Ease of identifying information	Uses a logical order to present information, with appropriate sub-headings and sections Utilises index page to aid location of relevant information Includes summary pages, where appropriate, to highlight key information Information and content clear, excellent images, font style and graphics	

Chapter 5

Frequently Asked Questions

Are DCT 1 posts available to general practitioners (associates) who may want to undertake further training?

DCT 1 posts are available to any individual who fulfils the DCT 1 national person specification. This may include those who have remained in practice setting following foundation training but decided to apply at a later date. If you are uncertain whether you can apply, you should email the designated contact on the application form and discuss your circumstances.

I've applied for a DCT post but did not get my preferred job – what shall I do?

DCT posts are varied, with each post offering different aspects of career progression. Depending on the area, there may be more posts in an OMFS department than a Dental Hospital post, but this does not make one more valuable than the other for the individual. It is important to research the posts you intend to apply for and understand your own personal development plan in order to come to an informed decision as to which post is best for you, rather than just go for the 'rare' posts.

Rejecting DCT training posts upon offer is also considered unprofessional and something that should not be done.

Will I get study days?

This will depend on the local trust/deanery arrangements and will form part of your contract. Many DCT jobs do have study days, and some deaneries will also offer a study budget, including paying towards conference fees and accommodation. Some deaneries will not provide locum cover and therefore you are not always guaranteed to be able to attend the study day.

If I begin DCT, but it is not for me, what do I do?

DCT posts are 12 months in duration; however, if you decide to leave earlier then this may affect your future DCT application.

Undertaking DCT 1 and leaving before the end of training may mean that your application is rejected for the subsequent year of DCT 1 application if you consider re-applying. The person specification states that to be eligible, you must

"Not have previously undertaken a Dental Core Training programme* or have completed less than 6 months of DCT 1 training by start date of post.

*If you are currently in or have previously undertaken a Dental Core Training year 1 post (or equivalent) but believe there are exceptional circumstances under which your application should be considered, you must detail this in the relevant section on your application."

It is essential you contact the DCTNRO early on to establish whether leaving your DCT post will impact your future position.

It is important to be proactive in your DCT post. You are in a salaried post and supported by a variety of consultants and lecturers with many opportunities, both clinical and non-clinical. Early in the year you should meet with your supervisor and discuss both your development plans and also how you can help the team you will be a part of. You have an allocated point of call should you have any concerns, but any decisions to leave a DCT year should not be taken lightly as not only will you have to declare this in future, but you may have denied a colleague a valuable learning experience. Do your research before!

Will I get a formal qualification after DCT?

There is no formal qualification, but the deanery will award a certificate of satisfactory completion. Successful completion of DCT 1 is required to advance forward to DCT 2, and the same is required for progression from DCT 2 to DCT 3.

Do I need to do DCT to specialise?

Having done a DCT 1 year, you will have demonstrated exposure to the management of complex cases within multidisciplinary teams. Working in different clinical environments often forms a part of the essential criteria of a specialist registrar person specification, and a DCT year will give evidence of this. However, there are many different specialties, and it is essential to be aware of their individual Person Specifications to help tailor your clinical (and non-clinical) experience. These can regularly be found on the Oriel website as and when specialty training posts are advertised.

One example of a desirable criterion for specialty training is 'Demonstrates the competencies required at the end of UK Dental Core training year 1 at the time of interview and year 2 at the time of post commencement (or equivalent).'

This demonstrates that DCT posts are valued in the selection of candidates for specialist training.

How many years of DCT do I need to do before I specialise?

See above. Different specialties will have different requirements, but the minimum postgraduate experience would be at least 3 years. This could include working in a variety of roles such as DCT (1 and 2), associate in general practice and staff grade. It would be highly recommended to read the person specification for specialty training for further details and contact the appropriate leads to guide decisions.

For those who are considering a specialist pathway in the future, an essential read is the Dental Gold Guide produced by COPDEND.

Can I get involved in teaching during DCT?

Yes, DCT is about being proactive and finding opportunities. This may include helping supervise students with consultants or carrying out group seminars/lectures. If this is something that interests you, you should contact your educational supervisor early in the year to help prepare some teaching experience. This is one of many valuable opportunities a DCT year can provide.

What if I have a disability – do I get extra time?

You must declare any disabilities at the application stage on the Oriel application form. You will also be required to email in and provide evidence of this disability. Health Education England policies outline the adjustments that can be made for individuals with a disability, and you will be informed of this before the assessment process.

Do I have to do MFDS or MJDF to get a DCT 1 post?

The DCT national person specification outlines that it is *desirable* for applicants to 'have a clear desire to pursue postgraduate qualifications.' Therefore, it is not essential; however, evidence of working towards or completion of any postgraduate award such as MJDF/MFDS or equivalent would be positively regarded.

Where in the career pathway is DCT?

Figure 2 illustrates the varied career path that a DCT may embark upon.

Figure 2. Dentistry career pathways beyond DCT 1

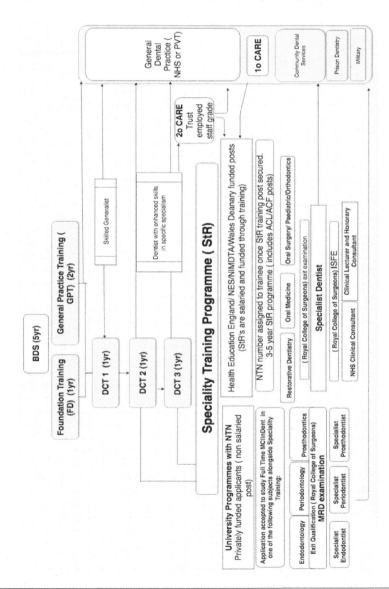

Figure 3. Restorative Pathways

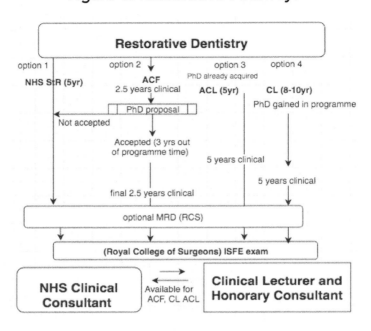

Option 1: NHS specialty training path is an NHS-funded route for trainees to gain specialist status. (60% clinical training, 25% academia, 15% research).

Option 2: NIHR Academic Clinical Fellowship post allows trainees to develop an aptitude for academia through research opportunities to support academic career progression. At the same time, the ACF will acquire the necessary clinical competencies required for entry onto the specialist list. (75% clinical training and 25% devoted to research). Successful ACF trainees will undertake a research project which may be funded by the affiliated University or via NIHR. Following completion of the 3-year fixed-term post, trainees may apply for an Out-of-Programme Research (OOPR) fellowship, allowing them to complete a higher degree (PhD).

Option 3: NIHR Academic Clinical Lectureship is available to dentists who wish to undertake specialty training and further research. General Dental Practitioners with a substantial amount of clinical experience may also be eligible for this role. (50% of time clinical training and 50% undertaking research or educational training).

Option 4: University-funded Clinical Lectureship is available to dentists who wish to develop research experience and pursue academia with subsequent specialty training. (50% of time clinical training and 50% undertaking research/educational training).

Figure 4. Oral Surgery/Paediatrics/Orthodontics

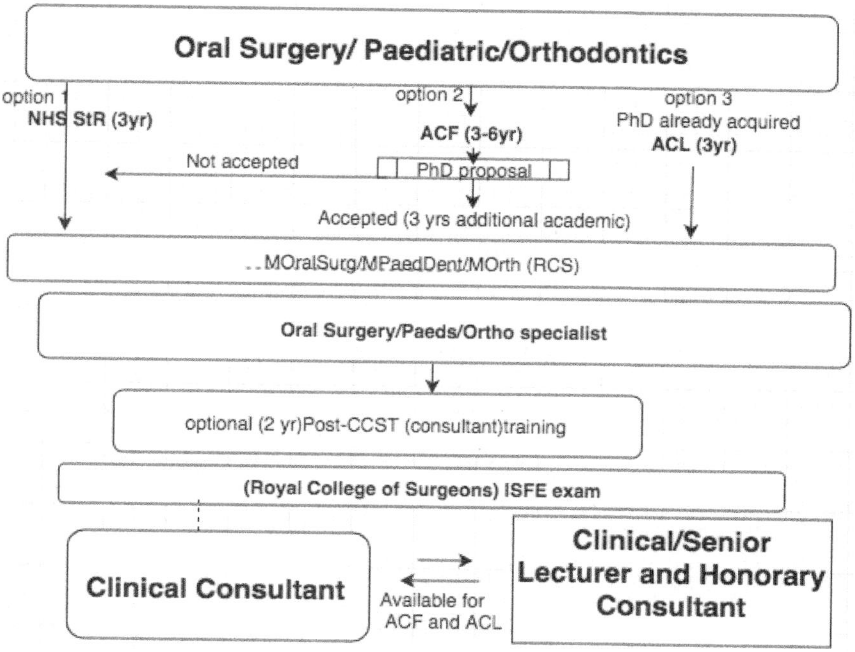

Option 1: NHS specialty training path is an NHS-funded route for trainees to gain specialist status. (100% clinical training). For job posts in certain regions and institutes, the length of post may vary, from a 3-year post to a 5-year run-through (a run-through post includes 3 years and a further 2 years post-CCST).

It is essential for you to read the information provided by the National Recruitment Office for your speciality of interest.

Option 2: NIHR Academic Clinical Fellowship post allows trainees to develop an aptitude for academia through research opportunities to support academic career progression. At the same time, the ACF will acquire the necessary clinical competencies required for entry onto the specialist list. (75% clinical training and 25% devoted to a research). Successful ACF trainees will undertake a research project which may be funded by the affiliated University or via NIHR. Following completion of the 3-year fixed-term post, trainees may apply for an Out-of-Programme Research (OOPR) fellowship, allowing them to complete a higher degree (PhD).

Option 3: NIHR Academic Clinical Lectureship is available to dentists who wish to undertake specialty training and further research. General Dental Practitioners with a substantial amount of clinical experience may also be eligible for this role. (50% of time clinical training and 50% undertaking research/educational training).

For more information with regards to Orthodontic Specialty Training, please see the British Orthodontic Society's document 'A guide to Applying for Orthodontic Training'.

https://www.bos.org.uk/Portals/0/Public/docs/Careers/AguidetoApplying_forOrthodonticTraining.pdf

Figure 5. Oral Medicine

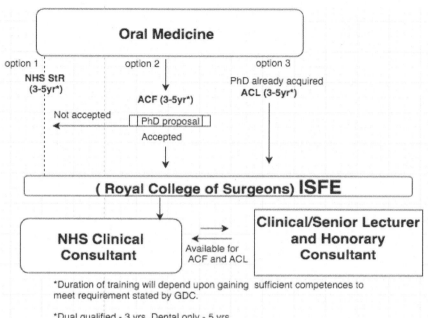

*Duration of training will depend upon gaining sufficient competences to meet requirement stated by GDC.

*Dual qualified - 3 yrs, Dental only - 5 yrs

Option 1: NHS specialty training path is an NHS-funded route for trainees to gain specialist status. (100% clinical training).

Option 2: NIHR Academic Clinical Fellowship post allows trainees to develop an aptitude for academia through research opportunities to support academic career progression. At the same time, the ACF will acquire the necessary clinical competencies required for entry onto the specialist list. (75% clinical training and 25% devoted to a research). Successful ACF trainees will undertake a research project which may be funded by the affiliated University or via NIHR. Following completion of the 3-year fixed-term post, trainees may apply for an Out-of-Programme Research (OOPR) fellowship, allowing them to complete a higher degree (PhD).

Option 3: NIHR Academic Clinical Lectureship is available to dentists and those who are dual (Medicine and Dentistry) qualified who wish to undertake specialty training and further research. General Dental Practitioners with a substantial amount of clinical experience may also be eligible for this role. (50% of time clinical training and 50% undertaking research/ educational training).

All applicants are strongly advised to read the post job description and person specification.

Figure 6. Mono-specialty pathway

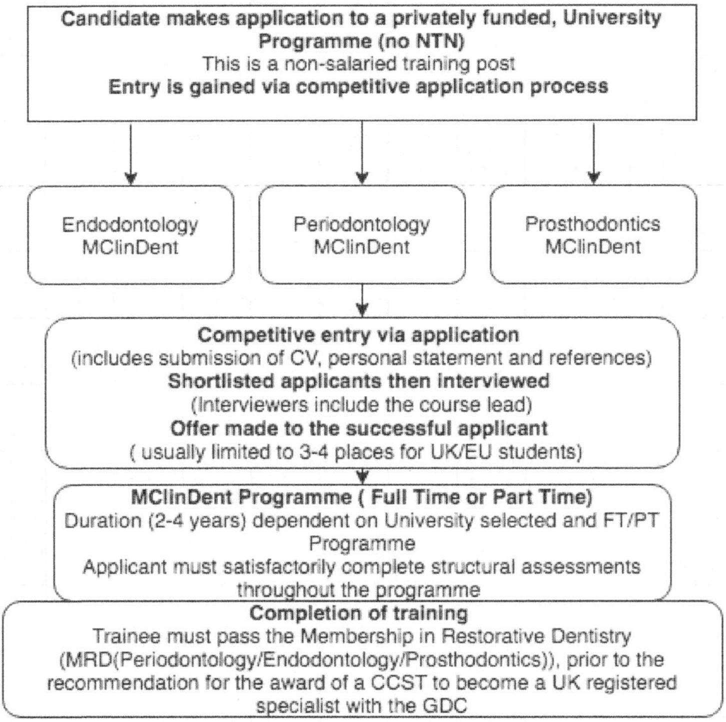

Candidate makes application to a privately funded, University Programme (no NTN)
This is a non-salaried training post
Entry is gained via competitive application process

Endodontology
MClinDent

Periodontology
MClinDent

Prosthodontics
MClinDent

Competitive entry via application
(includes submission of CV, personal statement and references)
Shortlisted applicants then interviewed
(Interviewers include the course lead)
Offer made to the successful applicant
(usually limited to 3-4 places for UK/EU students)

MClinDent Programme (Full Time or Part Time)
Duration (2-4 years) dependent on University selected and FT/PT Programme
Applicant must satisfactorily complete structural assessments throughout the programme

Completion of training
Trainee must pass the Membership in Restorative Dentistry (MRD(Periodontology/Endodontology/Prosthodontics)), prior to the recommendation for the award of a CCST to become a UK registered specialist with the GDC

Prior to 2018, certain Master of Clinical Dentistry (MClinDent) university programmes were assigned a National Training

Number (NTN). The provision of the NTN was previously gained via a competitive NHS Oriel recruitment process. This
allowed training dentists with an NTN to complete a university
higher degree (MClinDent Perio/Prostho/Endo) whilst gaining
competences required for entry onto the UK's GDC specialist
register, following passing the relevant membership examination for that particular speciality.

Since 2018, NTNs are no longer issued to those applying for
monospeciality training. Consideration of entry to the GDC
specialist list is now gained via mediation by the applicant achieving a recognised Master of Clinical Dentristy (MClinDent), the
relevant Royal College specialist diploma i.e. MPros, MPerio,
MEndo or MRD, and by satisfying the GDC with documented
portfolio of evidence.

The Authors

Dr Kalpesh Prajapat BDS (Liverpool), MFDS RCPS (Glasg)

Kalpesh graduated from Liverpool Dental School in 2016 with distinctions in Restorative Dentistry and Oral Health. Kalpesh was awarded several prizes both throughout undergraduate and during his early postgraduate career, with the most recent being the ADG postgraduate award in Dentistry. Following graduation, Kalpesh secured his first-choice foundation post in Cambridge. Kalpesh currently holds a DCT 2 post at Birmingham Dental Hospital in Sedation and Oral Surgery whilst also working part-time in general dental practice. Kalpesh secured his first-choice DCT 1 and 2 posts following the 2017 and 2018 national recruitment selection process. Kalpesh has interests in oral surgery, restorative dentistry, digital dentistry, and education.

Kalpesh was a key contributor to the DentaliQ interview preparation book for foundation training and also pioneered a bespoke SJT workshop in preparation for national recruitment foundation interviews. In addition, Kalpesh authored 'Dental Associate Interviews: An Ultimate Preparation Guide'; a guide for young clinicians embarking on the associate pathway.

Kalpesh was selected as one of the first UK dentists to join NHS England's Clinical Entrepreneur Fellowship programme aimed at bringing innovation into healthcare.

Dr Dima Mobarak BDS (Birm), MFDS RCPS (Glasg)

Dr Dima Mobarak graduated from The University of Birmingham in 2015. She has completed DCT 1 in Restorative Dentistry at Manchester Dental Hospital, DCT 2 in Oral & Maxillofacial Surgery in Birmingham and is currently in her DCT 3 year. She is passionate about education and is currently a mentor for younger dental students at her university. She has had a lot of experience in interview preparation having worked as an event coordinator with Dental Training Consultants, co-authored the DentaliQ book and App and organised DFT mock interview courses at national interview centres.

Dima is heavily involved in dental and non-dental humanitarian charity work, having set up oral health promotion schemes in local primary schools and trained junior Dentists in her projects. Outside of DCT, she works in private practice part-time and has presented at national and international conferences including the IADR in Seoul, Korea.